Accident & Emergency Nursing

A New Approach

Mike Walsh

BA SRN *Post-Grad. Cert. Ed.*
Charge Nurse in A & E
Royal Bristol Infirmary

Heinemann Nursing
London

ISBN 0–433–34820–8

© Mike Walsh 1985

First published 1985
by William Heinemann Medical Books Ltd
22 Bedford Square, London WC1B 3HH

Reprinted 1987

Photoset and Printed in Great Britain by
Redwood Burn Ltd., Trowbridge, Wiltshire

CONTENTS

ACKNOWLEDGEMENTS

I would first of all like to thank the staff of the West Cumberland Hospital, Whitehaven, who after giving me an immensely enjoyable training, launched me forth into the world of nursing with a great interest in A & E.

If the foundations for this book lie in the Cumbrian Fells, then the bricks and stone of which it is made originate with Barbara Vaughan and the staff of the Accident Service in Oxford where I did my JBCNS A & E Course. Bricks and stones need mortar to hold them together; the idea that patients are people needing individual understanding and nursing care is the mortar holding this book together. The ingredients for the mortar were the ideas learnt on the Diploma of Nursing at Bath Technical College, so to Helen Chalmers and the staff there—thank you for supplying the sand and cement!

Margaret Judd, Clinical Teacher in the School of Nursing of the Bristol Royal Infirmary, very kindly contributed the chapter on Women's Health Problems in A & E, and for this I am most grateful.

The staff of the Bristol Royal Infirmary A & E Unit deserve a special thanks for keeping me entertained over the past 6 years or so, making me several thousand cups of coffee, and putting up with my 5 a.m. cricket matches on night duty. A special thanks to the Ambulance Service, for without them doing their job properly out on the road, we would not be in business.

Turning to individuals, thanks to my mother and father and to Susan Florence and to Anne Kathryn. And special thanks to Maggy, Bethan, Ben, Boulmer and Hobo for making me smile again.

Finally I would like to thank the human race and hope that, despite the efforts of some politicians, we all still have a humane and caring future on this planet. After all, it is humanity and caring that this book is all about.

Mike Walsh
Bristol

PREFACE

This book has been spawned by the recognition that has grown up over the last ten years that Accident and Emergency nursing is a specialised branch of nursing in its own right. These last ten years have also seen the introduction into the UK of the nursing process and of the concepts of nursing as a profession that have been developed by American theorists such as Henderson, Roy and Orem. It is the aim of this book to bring together these strands of nursing theory and practice in such a way that the nurse who is new to the A & E department—be the nurse qualified or a student—can appreciate how care for each person can be optimised by treating that person in a holistic way, as a whole person, rather than as just 'the man with the leg in that cubicle there'.

In writing this book, I have tried to outline the bread and butter practice of A & E nursing, such as dealing with fractures, wounds and the common emergencies. But I have also tried to put into the picture the *person* whose leg is broken, whose arm is lacerated, whose coronary artery is thrombosed. If we are to practice the nursing process—the careful and logical planning, implementation, assessment and evaluation of care—we must appreciate our patient as a person with a mind and a social environment, both of which will influence the eventual outcome of our nursing efforts. So in writing this book, I have introduced sociology and psychology into the nursing care of the patient in the A & E department because it is only by taking these factors into account that can we give the best possible service to our clients as individuals.

In addition to the people with serious physical injuries and illnesses, there are many patients who attend A & E who are not so easy to help— the problem patients or so-called 'regulars', the drug overdosers, wrist slashers, drunks and vagrants, drifters and drug addicts, the flotsam and jetsam of our society. How can we deal with these people? Certainly there are no simple answers—but I hope that the reader may find the discussion of the care of these people, drawing as it does on sociology and psychology and practical A & E experience, a constructive section of the book.

Our patients or clients are people—individual people from individual different backgrounds with individual different thoughts and beliefs in their heads, not as of yet institutionalised by the hospital in-patient experience and routine. Let our nursing care, therefore, be individualised to each person—customised, if you like to think of it that way. I hope this book will encourage nurses in A & E to think of all their patients as individuals and to plan their nursing care in a logical problem-solving way based on this foundation. Remember, patients are people!

SECTION I

The Environment

Chapter 1

THE SOCIOLOGY OF TRAUMA AND ILLNESS

Each year 10 million people pass through the doors of A & E departments in the UK—a number approximately equal to the population of Australia. It can be said then that A & E nurses deal annually with a population equal to that of a major country. This implies that in their work A & E nurses will meet the full range of human society in terms of class, age, religion, ethnicity and culture. It is important, therefore, to place A & E nursing in its sociological perspective as it is from this extensive and varied tapestry of the human condition that our patients originate and to which we will return them.

In every tapestry, certain colours dominate and characteristic shapes and patterns are discernible as individual fibers are woven into the final complex picture. So it is with the sociological make up of a typical day's patients in an A & E department. There will be certain accident patterns that dominate (e.g. alcohol-related accidents, motorbike accidents, assaults) and the patterns will shift and change with the time of day. Furthermore, a large number of patients will have factors in common, such as occupation, age and class. These factors will give the A & E picture a characteristic social colouring. Looked at this way, therefore, A & E patients constitute a group from which striking sociological patterns emerge. These patterns demand the attention of the nurse if nursing care is to be carried out in the patient's best interest.

A discerning nose in A & E after 10 p.m. will detect the smell of alcohol on the breath of most patients. To what extent is alcohol a causative factor in trauma, especially late at night?

A glance through the register of any A & E department will show that certain districts or streets crop up with remarkable frequency. Is there a link between where people live and, therefore, their wealth, social class and their health record?

In looking through the register, it is quickly apparent that a high proportion of the patients are elderly, and that a high proportion of that group are elderly women requiring admission for fractures of the hip. What does that mean?

Imagine a line of over 1000 empty crash helmets, their owners all killed in the last 12 months. Think of a point two miles away and imagine a line of twisted and smashed motorbikes laid wheel to wheel stretching that distance; their riders will all have been seriously injured in the same 12 months that saw the death of 1000 of their comrades. What of these riders, is there anything unusual about their ages? Why are most of them men? Could it have to do with the aggressive/assertive conditioning of male children?

The woman with a bruised and battered face, the baby with a broken arm, the overdosed teenager having her stomach washed out, the junky on a bad trip and the depressed middle-aged alcoholic person are all familiar figures in A & E. They may seem to have very different problems, but could the root cause be the same? Could it be the breakdown and disintegration of normal family and interpersonal relationships?

The alert A & E nurse will quickly perceive these sorts of patterns. They represent only a few strands, however, of the sociological pattern that goes to make up A & E. Furthermore, while a tapestry is a permanent picture, A & E is a dynamic scene that changes with the passage of time in response to changes within society. The rest of this chapter will attempt to pick out some of these themes and patterns.

Accidents, Emergencies and Social Class

It is thought that there are two main causes of accidents—the environment and the behaviour of the individual. Both these causes are closely linked to social class. This link was explored as part of a much wider-ranging enquiry into health and society carried out under the chairmanship of Sir Douglas Black. This study, known as the Black Report, concluded that where you are in the social scale plays a major part in determining your health: '. . . gender and class exert highly significant influences on the quality and duration of life in modern society' (Townsend, Davidson, 1982).

One important finding of the Black Report was that, in the age range 16 to 64, the death rates for men of all social classes are nearly twice as high as the death rates for women. Clearly there are social forces at work that make being male in some ways more unhealthy than being female.

In order to see how mortality rates vary between social classes, and specifically how social class affects mortality due to accidents and emergencies, it is necessary to define social class. The definition chosen by the Black Report was that of the Registrar General which is based upon occupation.

Table 1.1

Registrar General's classification of social class by occupation and mortality

Class	Title	Mortality per 1000 pop age 16–64	
		Male	Female
I	Professional (e.g. lawyer, doctor)	3·98	2·15
II	Intermediate (e.g. nurse, teacher)	5·54	2·85
IIIN	Skilled non-manual (e.g. clerk, secretary)	5·80	2·76
IIIM	Skilled manual (e.g. carpenter, hairdresser)	6·08	3·41
IV	Partly skilled (e.g. postman/woman)	7·96	4·27
V	Unskilled (e.g. labourer, cleaner)	9·88	5·31

Source: *Occupational Mortality, England and Wales 1970–72*, HMSO 1978.

Table 1.1 gives mortality statistics according to social class and gender. It emerges clearly from this table that social class is a major determinant of health, with Social Class V having two and a half times the death rate of Social Class I. It should be noted that the figures in Table 1.1 pre-date the current recession and do not include the effects of unemployment. But if the gradient from I to V is extrapolated onwards to the even poorer unemployed then it is suggested that unemployment may be having a very deleterious effect on health indeed.

The mortality statistics relating to accidental death are shown in Fig. 1.1, and reveal a similar gradient, both for children and adults. The Standardised Mortality Ratio (SMR) is defined as the ratio of the numbers of deaths found to the numbers of deaths expected in a social class, allowing for the proportion of the total population found in that class. Thus an SMR of 100 is expected, while a ratio of over 100 is a worse than expected, and a ratio under 100 indicates a better than expected health record.

Figure 1.1 shows that social class exerts a major influence over the chances of any individual (child or adult) dying as a result of an accident. Children in Social Class V have over four times the likelihood of dying in accidents than children of Social Class I. Similar graphs to Fig. 1.1 can be plotted for other emergency conditions commonly seen in A & E such

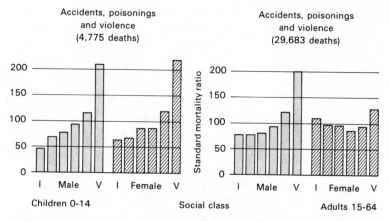

Fig. 1.1   Occupational class and mortality for children aged 0–14 and adults. (Source: Occupational Mortality, England and Wales 1970–72, HMSO, 1978.)

as cardiovascular, respiratory and genito-urinary diseases. The poorer social classes have the cards heavily stacked against them in terms of a more dangerous environment to live and work in, less health education, and fewer resources with which to look after their health.

This environmental effect is most clearly seen in the statistics for children, among whom in the UK and the rest of Europe, accidental death is the greatest single cause of death. Children in Social Class V have ten times the death rate from falls, fire and drowning, and five to seven times the death rate from road accidents than Social Class I children. Black states that 'While the death of a single child may appear as a random misfortune, this overall distribution indicates the social nature of the phenomenon'. Several factors can explain this difference: the lack of safe play areas in the poorer parts of towns and cities, the more dangerous types of household heating and furnishing which tend to be found in poorer homes, the lack of health knowledge among poorer groups, and the lack of parental supervision which is often due to situations where a single parent cannot take or is not granted time off from work to look after children who are on school holiday or off from school ill.

Social class determines where a person lives and to a significant degree the amount of stress in a person's life. There is plenty of evidence, in addition to the Black Report, to show how these factors affect the likelihood of a person becoming an A & E patient.

A survey by the Road Research Laboratory (1977) found that in urban areas where the housing dates from the 19th century, there is a road traffic accident rate two to three times greater than in areas of post-1919 housing, while the casualty rate among children from road accidents is twice as high in the areas of older type of housing than in the newer housing areas.

The effects of stress are shown by the work of Brown and Harris (1978) who studied mental health problems among working class women in Camberwell, London. Their conclusions were that 'The mother's psychiatric state and the presence of a serious long term difficulty or a threatening life event were related to increased accident risk to children under 16. These factors were more common among working class children and in so far as they are causal, they go a long way to explain the much greater risk of accidents to working class children'. Further evidence of the effects of the inner urban environment on child trauma comes from the work of Wilson and Herbert (1978) who carried out a detailed study of 56 families in deep poverty in central Birmingham. They found that in 34 of the families there had been serious accidents to children with one child losing an eye and 16 sustaining burns of such severity as to require skin grafting.

If criticism of the Black data is contemplated on the grounds that it relates to the early 1970s and is based on mortality statistics, then note should be taken of a survey carried out in 1984 in the A & E department at the Bristol Royal Infirmary (Walsh, 1984). This study revealed the same pattern of a marked class gradient for attendances. The only group which fared worse than Class V were the unemployed, unemployed women having the worst record of all. Non-utilisation of GPs was found to be very strongly class linked when the criteria used were that a patient should not attend A & E with an injury more than 12 hours old or with a complaint of non-traumatic nature (with certain obvious exceptions such as sudden chest pain or difficulty in breathing). Class V and the unemployed were found to have six times the attendance rates of Classes I and II and tended to have complaints that should more appropriately have been seen by GPs. This indicates a lack of knowledge among poorer people of how to use the health system, in particular their GPs.

Nurses are by definition Class II and are therefore likely to be from a different social class than that of many of their patients in A & E. But as individualised patient care can only be achieved by considering the social background of the patient, the nurse must be able and willing to bridge that social gap. In planning care the A & E nurse must be able to see the problem through the eyes of a single parent mother living on social security or a casual labourer who has lengthy spells on the dole in between jobs. Environment and class must be considered in nursing care as they affect the resources and health knowledge available to the patient on discharge from A & E. Patients are people and people are products of their environment, and it is that environment which is a major determining factor as to who attends A & E and why.

Age, Gender and Accidents

In writing his famous passage about the Seven Ages of Man in *As You Like It*, Shakespeare seemed to have one eye on a future A & E unit for A & E units span the whole human age range. In one cubicle there will be the person in 'second childishness and mere oblivion, sans teeth, sans eyes, sans taste, sans everything', while in the next cubicle will be 'the infant mewling and puking in nurse's arms'. This has significant implications for A & E nurses.

The increasing number of elderly people in our population, a result of demographic changes and increasing life span, has enormous implications for future health care demands, and A & E is not exempt from the effects of these trends. The elderly, because of failing faculties and other degenerative changes, are more prone to accidents. These accidents tend to have consequences which can be far more serious than in a younger person, particularly as they are often followed by major rehabilitative and social problems. One survey, for example, of fractures of the upper femur showed that the average age of victims of this serious injury was 82 (Walsh, 1984).

The high mortality rates in males under 65 (twice that of females) explains why in a recent survey in Bristol it was found that 16% of females presenting at A & E were over 70 years of age, while only 2.9% of male patients were. In the age range 16–64, however, there were twice as many male patients as female, while for children the ratio was only slightly less.

Road traffic accidents are undoubtedly a major factor in accounting for the high number of young people seen in A & E and the marked bias towards males. Table 1.2 shows that the vast majority of people who die or are seriously injured in RTAs are between the ages of 15 and 24.

The role of motorbikes in causing this tragic waste of young lives is well documented. Motorbikes are involved in more than eight times as many accidents as motor cars per mile travelled, resulting in the deaths of 1090 drivers and pillion passengers in 1982, compared to the deaths of 2443 car occupants, 1869 pedestrians and 294 cyclists in the same year.

Table 1.2
Age distribution of persons killed or seriously injured in RTAs 1982

Age	Number	Age	Number	Age	Number
0–4	1345	15–19	21 413	30–39	9366
5–9	3717	20–24	14 522	40–49	6250
10–14	5474	25–29	6964	50–59	5784
				60+	10 464

Source: Central Statistical Office (1982). *Annual Abstract of Statistics*.
London: HMSO.

A study into the cliché of 'women drivers' by Storie (1977) sheds some interesting light on the question of gender, accidents and their causes. Storie found no significant difference in accident rates between male and female car drivers, but she did find that twice as many men as women were driving too fast when they had their accident, and that men were far more likely to be involved in the overtaking accidents than females.

The much higher male attendance rate at A & E in the under 64 age group can be partly explained by the more hazardous nature of male work and sport. However, the tendency to aggression and assertiveness that is revealed by Storie's study undoubtedly underlies much male trauma leading as it does to more dangerous behaviour on the roads, increased alcohol consumption and violence. As male children are socialised into this aggressive/assertive role from childhood, nurses may speculate on how many accidents would be, in fact, preventable if we had different child rearing practices, and it should be remembered that the victims of male aggression are not always male.

Families, Women and A & E

Marxists see traditional families as a tool of capitalist oppression as they create a large pool of cheap female labour. Feminists, on the other hand, see families as trapping women and denying them equal rights. The traditional role of women in the family is under attack from all sides, and the trebling of the divorce rate between 1966 and 1976, one symptom of the changing role of women, has led to many women now being the lone heads of families. Of these lone mothers, only 18% are in full-time employment, although 78% have to cope with the burdens of living alone rather than with families.

In the many families where the woman is the head (104 524 divorces in 1982 had children), there are special problems when either the woman or her children become A & E patients. First, it is very difficult for a lone mother to supervise her children; the stress involved takes its toll on the mother—if she is ill, she may have to make special arrangements for someone to look after other young children, or the A & E unit will have to step into the breach on a temporary basis. Alternatively if one of the children is ill, the only way that the mother can accompany the child to A & E is to bring the rest of the children along as well. This requires that the A & E unit be able to look after well children as well as injured or ill children. Second, the lone mother is almost always confronted by the problem of poverty: only 18% have any full-time employment; for 34%, there are only part-time earnings, while for 48%, there are no earnings at all.

One further problem faced by women in the context of the family is that of violent partners. It is important for A & E nursing staff to realise that a woman's injuries may be due to violence from her partner, even though she may not admit this at first. A reluctance to leave the A & E unit after treatment for minor injuries suffered as a result of a 'fall' may be understood better in this light and A & E nurses should be alert for tell-tale signs of anxiety and inappropriate injuries when compared to the story of how they occurred. The existence of Women's Refuges should be known to the A & E nurse together with the knowledge of how to contact one if needed. A battered woman may be more prepared to talk about her problems to a female nurse than to a male doctor. She is most unlikely to involve the law. A study of battered women in Edinburgh reported that only 8% had taken legal action against their partners, despite 32% of the women reporting that assaults occurred as frequently as every week.

Another traditional role of the woman in the family is to look after aged relatives. However, increased family mobility, increased numbers of women in work, and the decline of the extended family have led to a decline in the numbers of women able to play this role. Elderly parents are left behind as their adult children move around the country. Distance weakens emotional ties; one week at Christmas does not compensate for 51 weeks apart and finally, after 20 to 30 years, children and parents may become strangers to each other.

A & E units face then a dual problem—an increasing number of elderly people living alone and who are therefore more accident prone, and fewer situations where an elderly patient can be discharged home with someone to look after them. Relatives of elderly patients who are unwilling to look after them (possibly for very good reasons) may feel very guilty, with the result that the wrong attitude by the nurse or an inadvertent word may lead to serious difficulty, which will be of no benefit to the patient and can lead to a serious deterioration in relationships between family and hospital. The A & E nurse should be non-judgemental at all times, and never more so than when dealing with the relatives of an elderly patient who refuse to take the patient home because they cannot look after him or her. The need is to see the problem from the family's perspective.

Culture, Ethnicity and A & E

The UK is fortunate in that it is a multiracial society and as a result has a rich and diverse cultural heritage and ambiance. If the A & E nurse is to give individualised patient care, then the ethnic and cultural background of the patient must be a major consideration. This in turn requires A & E nurses to familiarise themselves with cultural factors. It is a mistake for the nurse to judge the patient's beliefs against his or her own which will tend to be Caucasian Christian. Such an ethnocentric approach will lead to a failure in individualised care.

It is strange to talk of individualised care when many nurses do not know the patient's correct name, a situation that often arises with the Asian community. In the case of Sikhs, Singh merely indicates male and Kaur female; either title will be preceded by a personal name and followed by the name of the subcaste which is borne by the whole family (equivalent to a surname): for example, Mohinder Singh Sandhu or Gurmit Kaur Sondh would be correctly addressed as Mr Sandhu or Mrs Sondh. Sometimes the last name is dropped, and only then is it correct to talk of Mr Singh or Mrs Kaur. Hindus use one or more personal names followed by the subcaste name (equivalent to a surname) but do *not* use the titles Singh or Kaur.

The Muslim naming system is more complex as there are many titles that are not names, for example, Abdul, Mohammed, Shah, Syed; other titles such as Ahmad, Ahmed and Rahman can become names when combined with other titles, for example, Abdul Rahman. Khan and Choudhery are common names in Pakistan but these too are titles rather than names, while Bibi, Begum and Khatoon all signify that the bearer is female and do not act as true names. It is quite usual for members of the same family to have different names, with no common family name.

Human behaviour is largely learnt rather than innate, therefore the response to pain and illness will be environmentally determined. In other words, it will be a product of cultural background. This should lead the A & E nurse to realise that in dealing with patients from a different cultural background to the nurse, there will be significant differences in how the patient responds to illness and pain. Such differences are not to be interpreted as signs of weakness but rather as a normal learnt behaviour pattern. The whole concept of what is illness itself varies from ethnic group to ethnic group, and from class to class within any group. That which is defined as illness by one group may be considered normal by another, thus illness becomes socially constructed; its perception and how you respond to it are relative to where you are in society. Little is absolute!

Alcohol-related Accidents and Emergencies

Alcohol-related problems will be considered in depth later in the book. However, at this stage, the A & E nurse should recognise the role of alcohol as one of the major causative factors leading to the front door of A & E. The effects of alcohol on drivers is well known, but it is also a major factor in pedestrian trauma. A study in the West Midlands by Clayton, Booth and McCarthy (1977) found that 22% of all fatally injured pedestrians had a blood alcohol level above the legal limit for driving. At blood levels two and a half times the legal driving limit (about 5 pints of beer), the chances of being killed were 23 times greater than that of a control group. The social profile of the drink-impaired pedestrians who died was young to middle-aged, semi-skilled to unskilled (Social Class IV or V), divorced, separated or single.

There is an overwhelming volume of statistics which shows the effects of alcohol on drivers: Storie's survey found that alcohol was the greatest single impairment factor in accidents, that alcohol-impaired drivers were almost exclusively male, and that alcohol was involved in 35% of accidents where male drivers were to blame. Figure 1.2 shows how RTAs tend to occur around 11 p.m. to midnight, just after pubs close. Of these accidents, a third are fatal or cause serious injury.

Alcohol is frequently associated with acts of self-harm such as overdose and self-inflicted injury, while the depression of inhibition effect of alcohol leads to many acts of violence and other behaviour which terminates in trauma. The depression of inhibition may also result in behaviour which makes it impossible to treat a patient, and alcohol consumption will also delay the giving of an anaesthetic.

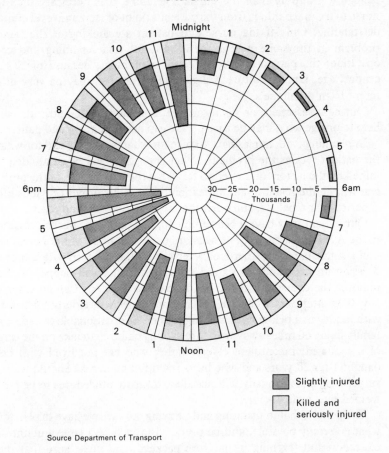

Slightly injured

Killed and
seriously injured

Source Department of Transport

*Fig. 1.2 Road accident casualties: by hour of the day and
severity of injury, 1982. (Source: Department of Transport.)*

The Nursing Process and Sociology

The first step in the nursing process is assessment. Social factors such as
class, age, gender, housing, and cultural and ethnic backgrounds will all
affect the A & E nurse's assessment of the patient. Furthermore,
without these factors being considered at all stages of the nursing process, there can be no individualised nursing care. This task is made more
difficult by the fact that often the patient will be from a very different so-

ciological grouping than the nurse. Therefore, it is necessary for the nurse to try to see things from the patient's point of view and level of understanding. Only if the nurse and patient are looking at the same problem in the same way is there hope for understanding and co-operation; the patient's perspective on a problem, because of class, gender, age, family, culture, religion and ethnicity, may be very different from the nurse's.

During assessment, an open-minded, non-judgemental attitude will help to bridge what may be a very wide gap between nurse and patient.

In planning care, nurses have to plan for what is possible and for what the patient sees as the problem. What is possible will be partly determined by the factors discussed so far; what the patient sees as the problem will be the result of an interaction between his or her previous life experience and beliefs, and what the nurse can explain and teach.

Our patient may have a beautifully applied plaster or burns dressing in the A & E department, but what are we sending him or her home to? Can a single parent mother look after two young children with a burns dressing on her hand? Does she understand what will happen if she removes the dressing and the hand becomes infected? Can an elderly lady look after herself (and her even more dependent elderly husband) with her leg in a below knee walking plaster? Is it reasonable to expect a family living 60 miles away with three young children to take on the care of a confused, incontinent elderly father who has not lived with his daughter for 20 years and who has a fractured humerus? Should we be surprised if an Asian lady will not allow intimate procedures to be performed by a male doctor?

The point is that in planning and carrying out care we have to plan for what is *socially* possible, and be prepared to include a large amount of education and teaching in our care package, and make sure that the patient understands fully the importance of what is being done. After all it is not what is taught that is important, it is what is learnt.

When we evaluate the success of our care, we must consider whether the goals set were socially attainable and realistic, and we must be prepared to alter our goals in accordance with experience and home environment.

In conclusion, the A & E nurse needs to realise how important environmental factors are in both the causation and care of the victims of trauma and sudden emergencies, and he or she needs to be prepared to take a leaf out of community nurses' book in giving due care and attention to the home and social circumstances of the patient.

Notes

1. In 1971 total new attendances at A & E departments in the UK were 9 358 000. By 1981 that figure had risen to 11 342 000.
2. Mortality rates per thousand population for 1982 were as follows:

Age	Male	Female	Ratio	Age	Male	Female	Ratio
0–4	3·2	2·5	1·28	20–24	0·9	0·4	2·25
5–9	0·3	0·2	1·50	25–34	1·0	0·5	2·00
10–14	0·3	0·2	1·50	35–44	2·0	1·3	1·54
15–19	0·9	0·3	3·00	45–54	6·4	3·9	1·64
				55–64	19·3	10·0	1·93

Road traffic accidents are probably a major cause of the fact that teenage males are three times more likely to die than teenage females. Source: *CSO Annual Abstract of Statistics*. London: HMSO. 1984.

References and Further Reading

Brown G., Harris T. (1978). *The Social Origins of Depression*. London: Tavistock.

Clayton B., Booth A. C., McCarthy P. E. (1977). *A Controlled Study of the Role of Alcohol in Fatal Adult Pedestrian Accidents*. Transport and Road Research Laboratory.

O'Neil P. (1983). *Health Crisis 2000*. London: Heinemann Medical Books.

Storie V. J. (1977). *Male and Female Car Drivers, Differences Observed in Accidents*. Transport and Road Research Laboratory.

Townsend P., Davidson N. (1982). *Inequalities in Health*. Harmondsworth: Penguin.

Wilson H., Herbert G. W. (1978). *Parents and Children in the Inner City*. London: Routledge, Kegan & Paul.

Walsh M. (1984). *Social Class and Attendances at A & E in Bristol*. (unpublished).

Chapter 2

PATIENTS, PEOPLE AND NURSES— PSYCHOLOGY IN A & E

This chapter could be subtitled 'Hearts and Bones' because there is more to A & E nursing than physical problems such as broken bones. There are emotional and mental problems as well. An understanding of psychology is essential for good nursing practice for how can we truly individualise care unless we consider the mental processes of our patients? This chapter aims, therefore, to familiarise the reader with some of the areas of psychology that are most relevant to A & E and to show how psychological insights can make a real and beneficial impact on patient care.

Emotion

In A & E nurses work in an emotion-charged atmosphere. They come into contact with depression and sadness, happiness and joy, and guilt and anger—in fact, with the full range of human emotion. The suddenness with which many patients are taken ill and the media image of the A & E department—as a place full of wailing sirens, flashing blue lights and life-saving heroics—combine to make sudden illness in the A & E department a highly emotional and anxiety provoking experience for the general public.

Nurses sometimes overlook the emotional content of a patient or a relative in A & E, because they do not know what they are looking for. However, there is a useful body of research on the psychology of emotion that can be applied to the A & E department to improve nursing care and to prevent problems arising out of emotional behaviour.

The key work in the field of emotion is that of Stanley Schachter and his co-workers. Schachter (1962) showed that emotion consists of three parts. First, there is an external event that stimulates the autonomic nervous system leading to our arousal, but in a non-differentiated and generalised way. Two other factors then convert this general arousal into a specific emotion that we recognise as anger or fear. Schachter's experiments showed that these key factors are cues provided by the environment and our previous experience of similar events. Emotion, Schachter therefore concluded, consists of three components: arousal, environmental cues and previous experience.

The sudden onset of illness or trauma followed by the rapid movement to A & E will certainly act as an emotionally arousing event leading to autonomic stimulation. Similarly, when a family is told that their relative has been 'rushed to hospital', their emotions will be aroused.

When the patient and the family arrive in the A & E, together or apart, the nurse will be one of the most potent sources of emotional cues. Schachter's work suggests that much of the patient's emotional behaviour will depend on the nurse's behaviour. If the nurse is anxious and hostile, the patient may well be anxious and hostile. Conversely, if the nurse is calm and confident, this manner will help bring a distressed patient to a clearer and calmer state of mind. The same applies to the nurse's interaction with the family.

In addition, nurses should remember the effect of previous experience on emotion and consider that a patient's apparently unreasonable emotions may have their origins in some previous unhappy experience. Furthermore, as today is tomorrow's yesterday, the experience undergone by patients today will have an important effect on their reaction to future hospitalisation; this is especially true of young children and their fears of hospital.

In short, A & E patients are emotionally aroused and will tend to take cues which will affect those emotions from what they see around them. Control the emotional environment (including the nursing staff's emotions) and the patients' and families' emotions will be largely controlled.

Grief and Bereavement

Today some two-thirds of all deaths occur in institutions, with a high proportion of sudden deaths occurring in A & E departments. It is the suddenness of death in A & E and the age range involved that makes coping with death and the bereaved family and friends one of the most difficult aspects of A & E work.

Most nurses will have witnessed death before coming to A & E, but these deaths will usually have been the result of a lengthy illness so that the act of dying is expected and fits well into Saunders' moving description of terminally ill patients (1959).

They were not frightened nor unwilling to go, for by then they were too far away to want to come back. They were conscious of leaving weakness and exhaustion rather than life and its activities. They rarely had any pain but felt intensely weary. They wanted to say goodbye to those they loved but were not torn with longing to stay with them.

In contrast, the dead person in the A & E department is unfortunately but often the cheerful child last seen by his mother setting off to school, the baby found in its cot, the husband and father collapsing at work or the teenager who never came home from a party. It is the stunning suddenness of this most final act of all that lends such a devastating dimension to the problem of caring for the bereaved in A & E.

The grief reaction consists of a cultural and an individual component. Nurses in A & E should remember that the cultural background of the bereaved may be very different from their own and, therefore, not to be surprised if the relatives' behaviour is different from that which nurses expect as a result of their own cultural upbringing (Parks, 1972; Smith, 1978).

Hinton's description of grief (1972) includes shock, denial, anxiety, depression, guilt, anger and a wide range of somatic signs linked to anxiety. However, these manifestations should not be thought of as a strict succession of stages. Regression is also common.

It is a long walk from the resuscitation room to the relatives waiting room when a patient has died. How can the above comments help the nurse who has to make that walk with bad news to impart at the end? The response of relatives will vary with culture and individual factors, therefore their response may lie anywhere in a wide range of behaviours—from stunned unbelieving silence through to collapse and a flood of emotion and on to stoical acceptance. The nurse should not be fooled by the stoical response, for whatever the response, the grief is there and it has to be worked through in the long term. Stoicism certainly does not convey a lack of care for the dead person or an easy acceptance of the death.

The nurse must be prepared for many questions. 'Why me?' 'Why her?' 'Couldn't anything be done?' 'Its all my fault, isn't it?' These questions do not have answers in this context. A denial response may be observed with the relative simply refusing to believe the person is dead. This denial has to be overcome as an essential part of the grief work, if acceptance is to be reached. The relative should be shown the body and allowed to touch and feel the deceased in order to help with the grief work. This is especially true of mothers of children and infants who have died (particularly cot death infants). The mother should be encouraged to hold the dead baby in her arms to help her overcome the denial mechanism so that she may more readily come to terms with the death of her baby.

A single bereaved person should never be left alone in the department or left to go home alone. Somebody must sit with them until a relative or friend can be found. Providing human company at this most difficult hour of a person's life is a nursing responsibility. In providing that company, nurses provide the person with an opportunity to verbalise their grief and they protect the person from possible harm. If in the process of doing this, nurses themselves feel moved to tears, there is nothing wrong in that. It is an expression of human empathy, not inadequacy.

One important practical point concerns the identification of the deceased. Friends can mistakenly identify a person they have known for years under the stress of an A & E resuscitation room and in the aftermath of a resuscitation attempt on a badly injured patient. The result may be that the wrong relatives are informed.

If nurses find that they are upset by a death in A & E, they should know that this is a normal reaction to a very stressful event that is rather different from death in other hospital areas. Nurses in A & E can take comfort in the fact that although sometimes we do lose a life, there are times when we win as well. And most of the time, our work lies somewhere in between—we simply help people through their present problems.

How We Perceive Others

How do patients perceive nurses and how do nurses perceive patients? Research into person perception suggests that the answer may be that they perceive each other very differently and that neither's perceptions may be very accurate. Nurses need to look carefully at how misperception occurs, for misperception may radically alter their assessment of the patient—and accurate assessment is central to the process of nursing.

One view of perception sees it as depending heavily upon previous experiences, with judgements being inferred from the information available. In addition, however, we have systems of rules by which we understand what we perceive. These association rules are based on experience and culture. Some may in addition be unique to the individual. These rules create mental sets that act as pigeon holes into which perceived information can be conveniently filed and rapidly understood.

The formation of association rules in this way unfortunately leads us on to form stereotypes to which we consign people. Stereotyping is a common human perceptual process, but it is frequently wrong. In A & E we will meet all manner of people from all walks of life and from different cultural and religious backgrounds; we would be making a serious error if we were to let stereotyping govern our assessment. We must look beyond the clothes and other outward appearances and assess the person underneath objectively and individually rather than consign him or her to a stereotype as 'a typical . . .'.

Another interesting aspect of human perception is described by Jones and Davis (1965). They showed that the more abnormal a person's behaviour is, the more likely we are to attribute the reason for that behaviour to something within the person rather than to the environment which could be equally responsible. Is it not possible that some of the strange behaviour that we see in A & E and readily assign to the patient, could more easily be understood in terms of a reaction to the A & E environment rather than something wrong within the patient?

In the first chapter, nurses were reminded that they are nurses not judges and they should not sit in judgement on their patients. Experiments by Waltster (1966) have shown that when we judge someone to be guilty, we are more influenced by the results of an act than by the act itself. How do we feel about the drunken driver who has lost control of his car, crashing it and killing a young child in the process, compared to the equally drunk driver who crashed his car but suffered only minor injuries to himself? The act is the same—drunken driving—but the very different results tend to lead us to very different judgements. This underlines the minefield that lies in wait for A & E nurses who start to judge their patients.

The hedonistic principle described by Jones and De Charms (1964) describes how if a person's actions interfere with our own pleasure, we view them in a less favourable light. Therefore, it is not a good idea to ask a nurse to make an assessment 5 minutes before he or she is due to go off duty. The nurse's assessment may be negatively affected.

One final aspect of perception is the old cliché that 'first impressions count'. Luchins (1957) carried out research which showed that there is a great deal of truth in this statement. In forming impressions of people, we do allow our first impression to control much of what follows, often leading to serious errors in perception. If A & E nurses are aware of this trap, they will find it easier to put first impressions to one side and to spend time talking to patients, trying to get to know them a little better, before making an assessment. Their assessment will be more accurate for the time spent.

It should also be remembered that the same mechanisms which cause misperception are also at work in the patient. He will be working with a stereotype of you as a nurse. He will tend to form an impression of you based on the first minute of your interaction. He will tend to judge you by the results of your actions rather than by the actions themselves. Furthermore, if your actions interfere with his pleasure, do not be surprised if your ratings drop accordingly, despite the fact that what you are doing is in the patient's interests in the long run.

In short, if the A & E nurse is to make an accurate assessment of the patient, there is a need to be aware of the range of factors which influence human perception.

How We Perceive our Environment— Sensory Deprivation in A & E

When a person is deprived of meaningful sensory input, they are said to be experiencing sensory deprivation. Experimental work has shown that, after a period of only a few hours, sensory deprivation can produce hallucinations, anxiety, fear and other mental disturbances.

Let us think of a typical A & E cubicle where a patient can remain for several hours. What sensory input does a patient have in that situation? There is no clock to tell the time. Often the patient cannot even tell if it is day or night. The walls are blank. Loose curtains block off the view beyond the end of the trolley. Overhead there is the ubiquitous neon strip lamp in an equally bare ceiling. If the patient has no friends or relatives present, and no nurse has the time to chat with her, how will she be able to assess the passage of time? We have put our patient into a state of sensory deprivation. How much apparent 'confusion' in elderly patients starts in the environment of sensory deprivation that we subject our patients to in the A & E cubicle? To take the case a step further, what if the patient is deaf or wears spectacles and the hearing aid or spectacles are at home? The sensory deprivation will be even more acute.

The patient will probably also be suffering from perceptual deprivation as we may be exposing her to stimuli that are meaningless: the x-ray machines, the ECG monitors, the strange sounds and the mysterious jargon of modern hospitals mean very little to most people. All this adds up to the patient being deprived of meaningful perceptions.

Many sudden mood changes and cases of apparent confusion, therefore, are probably the result of the A & E environment depriving the patient of meaningful sensations and perceptions. If a patient is likely to be in A & E for any length of time, reality orientation must be a vital part of the care plan. Leave the curtain at the end of the cubicle pulled back a little so patients can see what is going on. Tell them the time. Talk to them. Make sure spectacles and hearing aids are worn and working. Explain the sounds and sights of the A & E department so that patients have meaningful perceptions of it (the nurse as the interpreter of the hospital experience). Above all, give the patients some meaningful stimulation. Nurses may even want to consider having quiet piped radio in the A & E to help while away the time.

In short, A & E nursing staff need to be aware of the risks of sensory deprivation to their patients.

Learning and Behaviour

Why do we behave the way that we do? This is a question that has exercised the minds of many famous philosophers and scientists; it is also a question that has a great deal of relevance to the work of A & E nurses. One way of looking at this question comes from the Behaviourist School which had its origins in the experiments of Thorndike and Skinner in the early years of this century.

The main thrust of behaviourism is that human behaviour is a product of learning experiences and of the environment and that it is not due to pre-programmed activity or instinct. This implies, therefore, that behaviour can be learned and can be changed. As nurses, we often need to do just that, change behaviour. Hence the importance of behaviourism to learning—and to nursing care.

Let us first of all consider learning through operant conditioning. If an act is followed by desirable experiences, it is more likely to be repeated; the desirable consequences act as positive reinforcement. If an act is followed by punishment, the effect is to suppress the behaviour, but not to eliminate it—for when the punishment is removed, the behaviour will reappear.

A more effective way of eliminating behaviour is by *extinction*. In this case, positive reinforcement is withheld. This leads to a long-term removal of the behaviour.

These three ideas can be illustrated with a familiar example in A & E. A disturbed young woman with a disordered personality is a regular attender at A & E. She comes in regularly with self-inflicted minor lacerations on the arms, accompanied by attention-seeking and disruptive behaviour. The attention that follows such actions acts as a positive reinforcement leading to repetition of this behaviour. If, however, the attention that the woman receives and the disruption that she causes with each visit are denied to her—if we simply ignore her behaviour—then the extinction effect will be expected to lead to the patient discontinuing her self-harming and attention-seeking behaviour. On the other hand, a punitive response—for example, calling the police to remove the patient—will lead to further disruption and more positive reinforcement. In the long run, court proceedings will not usually have much effect on this sort of situation.

Nurses with personal experience of this sort of situation vouch for the efficacy of the extinction principle in controlling disruptive behaviour. The punitive approach simply rewards the patient with attention that they want and leads to more disruptive behaviour.

A further form of learning that comes under the heading of operant conditioning is negative reinforcement. In this case, behaviour leads to the removal of unpleasant or adverse situations. Alcohol abuse is a good example of negative reinforcement; the patient drinks to avoid the difficult realities of everyday life. Some of the difficult behaviour of elderly patients can be also explained in terms of avoiding problems of living by getting other people to perform various tasks for them.

Positive reinforcement is potentially a powerful tool for the nurse who seeks patient compliance and for the nurse who wants to teach and motivate junior staff. In teaching a patient how to use crutches or how to do the essential finger exercises for an arm in plaster, we must reward correct actions with praise (positive reinforcement) if we want those actions to be repeated. Similarly, if a junior member of staff is being taught a skill or a junior nurse performs an intelligent or thoughtful piece of nursing care, then we should praise the nurse and say 'well done'. Such positive reinforcement will produce a more caring, better motivated and more skilful nurse. Ignoring good work will produce extinction of that good work. While merely telling the nurse off for poor work (punitive reinforcement) will not bring about good care.

Having discussed operant conditioning, it now remains to look at classical conditioning, the origins of which lie in the famous work of Pavlov and his dogs (Fig. 2.1). Pavlov presented food to a dog (unconditioned stimulus) and obtained a response of salivation (unconditioned response) which was a reflex action. If he rang a bell at the same time (conditioned stimulus), he found that after a while the dog associated the bell with the food and salivated to the sound of the bell only. Salivation had become a conditioned response.

This form of learning has been demonstrated in humans. Consider the

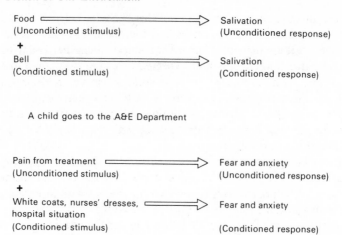

Fig.2.1   *Pavlov's classic experiment and an A & E example: the unconditioned and conditioned stimulus become paired together to produce a conditioned response.*

example of the small child taken to A & E after an accident. The combined efforts of the nurses and a casualty officer may do a very good job of stitching his scalp back together, but this can be a very frightening experience for the child. The strange environment and those funny strangers in white coats and dresses will become associated with the pain and discomfort involved in having a wound stitched. The result will be that the next time the child has to attend hospital, white coats and nurses' dresses will act as a conditioned stimulus to produce the conditioned response of fear and anxiety. It is thought that the origins of many irrational fears and phobias lie in this mechanism, where the response to one stimulus is transferred onto another stimulus by classical conditioning. Examples range from fear of injections through to phobias about spiders and on to sexual fetishes.

The implications of Pavlov's work for the A & E nursing of children is clear: if we want to prevent children developing fears about hospitals, the unconditioned stimulus must be minimised by reducing pain and discomfort to a minimum; children's experience of A & E must be made as least unpleasant as possible; on the other hand, we can also try to remove the conditioning stimulus of white coats, nurses' uniforms and all the other hospital paraphernalia. Ideally there should be a special children's section in the A & E department with toys and a play area, where staff should be in mufti and where the hospital environment should be minimised as far as possible.

One final method of learning behaviour that needs discussion is learning by imitation. Bandura (1973) showed that children learn violent behaviour by copying adults. In nursing, more senior nurses act as models for junior staff all the time; imitation or modelling has been shown to be a very potent way of learning practical skills. Student nurses are often caught in a dilemma, being taught to do a nursing procedure one way in the school and then seeing it done very differently in practice. The power of modelling as a means of learning behaviour is so potent that where different methods are taught, it is not surprising that the student copies what he or she has seen in the clinical setting and that the procedure taught as theory in the school rarely translates into practice. A great deal of student unhappiness could be avoided by schools of nursing and service areas such as A & E coordinating their teaching much more closely.

Memory

How do we remember information? What can we do to improve recall? These two questions deserve our attention if we are to ensure optimum results from teaching patients prior to discharge about their dressings, exercises, plasters and other aspects of care. If a patient fails to take adequate care of his plaster and if he forgets the importance of tingling and discoloration in his fingers and of exercising his fingers, the patient who was sent home with a straightforward Colles fracture treated with a standard plaster of Paris may experience serious complications. Similar comments apply to a whole range of treatments, drugs and instructions with which we discharge patients every day from A & E. Nurses, therefore, need to know something of the work that has been done in the field of memory for not only will it benefit patients, but incorporated into teaching, it will improve the way that student nurses learn.

Insights into memory can be gained from the work of Murdock (1962). He gave people a series of words to remember and later tested them to see which could be recalled. The results were plotted as a serial position curve as shown in Fig. 2.2. On this graph, the frequency of successful recall of any word is plotted against its position in the series of words given.

The curve that Murdock plotted can be explained as follows. Memory is thought of as consisting of two components, long-term memory (LTM) and short-term memory (STM). The short-term part of memory can only retain about seven items which are then either lost from STM

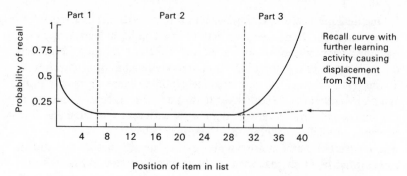

Fig. 2.2.   Free recall curve. (Murdock 1962, Glanzer 1972)

by displacement by new items to remember or are passed on into LTM after appropriate rehearsal. If we study the curve, it becomes apparent that the high success rate at the end of the curve (Part 3) is due to short-term memory. However, if we give the person another learning activity to perform immediately afterwards, the effect is to greatly reduce the recall (dashed line) due to items being displaced out of short-term memory by the new learning activity.

The high success rate in Part 1 of the curve reflects the working of LTM and is called the primacy effect. However, LTM will diminish (Part 2) due to emotional upset and interference, where similar items get in the way of what we are trying to recall. Improvements in LTM can be brought about by repetition of what is to be remembered and by the pro-vision of cues to enable us to access information more readily in LTM.

How then can the A & E nurse apply some of these insights into memory to improve care? Murdock's work shows us that a patient will recall best what is said first and last. Therefore, we must put the most important information first and last. To help patients to remember what is said in the middle (and there has to be a middle), we can use repetition of key points coupled with cues to help memory; at the same time, we should try to avoid introducing spurious information which will only interfere with what has to be remembered, especially if it is similar in content. Emotional upset will interfere with memory also, so there is not much point expecting someone who is very anxious or distressed to remember detailed instructions—their emotional state has to be stabil-ised first. Finally, given the fallibility of human memory, consideration should be given to simple pre-printed instruction cards for such things as care of plaster of Paris, wounds, anti-tetanus follow-up and so on.

The points made in this section can be applied with equal validity when considering how best to help student nurses to remember what they have been taught.

Language Codes—
Do Nurses and Patients Speak the Same Language?

There is a substantial body of research that suggests that there are different forms of English in use, known as codes, and that these codes are class-related (Bernstein, 1961, 1973; Hawkins, 1969). If patient and nurse are using different codes or different forms of language, then there is a real risk of inadequate communication and misunderstanding between them.

Researchers postulate that there are two forms of language, elaborated code (typically middle class) and restricted code (typically working class). They are differentiated by the fact that elaborated code is grammatically more complex and uses a richer content of adjectives than the restricted code. This results in the meaning of an elaborate code sentence being said to be explicit or spelt out. The meaning of a restricted code sentence, on the other hand, is implicit or not spelt out. The consequence is that one restricted code user may understand what is implicitly meant by another restricted code user, but an elaborate code user who is used to a much more explicit use of English may fail to understand what is being said. Because of their educational backgrounds, nurses are often elaborate code users. The elaborate code of the middle-class nurse, grammatically complex and with a large number of adjectives, may prove overwhelming to a patient who uses restricted code English. This problem of understanding which stems from different uses of English between patient and nurse is exacerbated by the use of technical jargon that few people outside the medico-nursing world can understand.

In summary then, when talking to patients and in particular when obtaining a history or giving self-care instructions before discharge, the nurse needs to be aware of the potential for different uses of English and of the misunderstandings that can ensue from different codes. Many nurses are from a middle-class background (although many are not) and they need to be aware that there is a different use of language by their working-class patients which may make the task of obtaining a history, for example, rather more difficult than would have been imagined due to the meanings in the patients' language that are buried away from the nurses' comprehension. How often do we see the phrase 'poor historian' written in medical notes? The patient's meanings would probably be quite clear to another restricted code user who would grasp the implicit meanings behind the limited use of vocabulary.

The reverse situation applies when the nurse is seeking to pass information to the patient: nurses need to talk in language that the patient understands and to make it simple if the patient is using a restricted code. However, oversimplification of instructions to elaborate code users may make them feel that they are being patronised and they will resent this.

Patient assessment should include a mental assessment of the type of language code used by the patient, so that the nurse can communicate well.

The Psychology of Ageing

Important psychological changes occur with ageing, both in childhood and old age. A discussion of these changes has been left, however, to the relevant chapters later in the book which look at the problems of children and the elderly in the A & E department.

The Nursing Process and Psychology

It remains to try to pull together some of the aspects of psychology touched upon in this chapter and show their importance to the nursing process in A & E.

If we start at the assessment stage, we are largely involved with obtaining information from and about the patient. The ease with which an assessment interview is conducted, and to some extent, the physical signs that are displayed (for example, pulse and blood pressure) will be affected by the emotional state of the patient. We have already seen that nurses can act as a major controlling influence upon emotion by the cues they provide to the emotionally aroused patient and relatives. Some knowledge about human perception should make the nurse aware of the pitfalls that lie in wait for us in our perception of others: nurses need to beware stereotypes and first impressions, take into account the patient's environment and its likely effect upon his or her behaviour, and avoid the temptation to make judgemental assessments. Finally, the nurse should remember that people have different ways of using English depending upon their class background with the result that a meaning that may be perfectly clear to the nurse may be completely baffling to the patient. The reverse situation also applies.

In planning patient care, there is a need to consider how best to avoid creating fears and phobias, especially in children, by inadvertent classical conditioning. The use of behaviourist techniques such as positive reinforcement and extinction should be considered in modifying behaviour both with staff or patients. In planning for maximum recall of information, the various aspects of memory theory have an important place. One final area of planning where psychological knowledge is of importance is in planning for the care of bereaved relatives.

A major problem in the implementation of nursing care is pain, which in turn is greatly affected by psychological factors. Pain is more than just a simple response to tissue damage; it is an experience born of the person's response to that damage but greatly influenced by the perception of the situation that the person is in. Thus anxiety, fear, depression, cultural background and expectations are all factors that have been shown to influence the degree of pain that a person experiences. Nursing intervention to allay fear and anxiety and to explain what is likely to happen next to the patient will make a great contribution to the reduction of pain as experienced by the patient. We can thus see that much of the research mentioned in this chapter into areas such as emotion and perception have great relevance in implementing nursing care around the goal of reducing pain.

In evaluating the effectiveness of our nursing interventions, we need to take into account again the misperceptions and language problems that can arise from code usage being different in patient and nurse, as well as from the 'jargon-speak' that the patient cannot understand. Evaluation of the effectiveness in pain reduction must take into account differences of culture—it would be a mistake to judge non-Europeans by European standards, or South Europeans by North European standards and so on.

This chapter has looked at some of the aspects of psychology that may allow the A & E nurse to see patients in a different light, and to understand better the sometimes odd ways in which people behave when under the twin stresses, on the one hand, of acute illness and pain and, on the other hand, of the strange and unfamiliar environment of hospital. It is not the nurse who is ill and to the nurse the hospital is a familiar environment. It is from this dysjunction of experience that many problems arise in A & E that could be resolved with a little consideration of the psychological processes involved.

References and Further Reading

Emotion
Schachter S., Singer J. E. (1962). Cognitive, Social and Physiological Determinants of Emotional States. *Psychological Review*, **69**: 379–99.

Grief
Hinton J. (1972). *Dying*. Harmondsworth: Penguin.
Kübler-Ross E. (1973). *On Death and Dying*. London: Tavistock.
Saunders C. (1959). *Care of the Dying*. London: Macmillan.
Parks C. M. (1972). *Bereavement: Studies of Grief in Later Life*. London: Tavistock.
Smith K. (1978). *Help for the Bereaved*. London: Ducksworth.

Perception
Bandura K. (1973). *Aggression: a Social Learning Analysis*. Englewood Cliffs, NJ: Prentice-Hall.
Jones E. E., Davis K. E. (1965). From acts to dispositions. In *Advances in Experimental Social Psychology*, **2**: 219–66 (Berkowitz L., ed.). New York: Academic Press.
Jones E. E., De Charms R. (1957). Changes in social perception as a function of the personal relevance of behaviour. *Sociometry*, 75–85.
Luchins A. (1957). Primacy-Recency in Impression Formation. In *The Order of Presentation in Persuasion* (Houland C. I., ed.). New Haven: Yale University Press.
Murdock B. B. (1962). The Serial Position Effect in Free Recall. *Journal of Experimental Psychiatry*, **65**: 482–6.
Walster E. (1966). The Assignment of Responsibility for an Accident. *J. Pers. Soc. Psychol.*, **5**: 508–16.

Language
Bernstein B. (1961). Aspects of Language and Learning in the Genesis of the Social Process. *J. Child Psychology and Psychiatry*, **1**: 313–24.
Bernstein B. (1973). *Class Codes and Control*. London: Paladin.

General Reading
Hilgard E., Hilgard R., Atkinson R. C. (1979). *Introduction to Psychology*. New York: Harcourt Brace Jovanovich Inc.

Chapter 3

THE ROLE OF THE NURSE IN A & E

Nye Bevan, the man thought of as the founding father of the NHS, once said that the only difference between a rut and a grave was that one was deeper than the other. Traditional nursing practice has worn a large number of ruts, some of which must be very deep by now, and A & E nursing is probably not exempt from wearing ruts. However, if we wish to prevent ruts from turning into graves containing a nursing practice that is lifeless, then nursing needs to think anew about its role and rationale.

The aim of this chapter is to explore some new ways of looking at nursing and how such ideas can be of use in the A & E department.

Models of Nursing and their Application in A & E

Any profession must have well-established theoretical foundations. Nursing is no exception to this rule and vague notions about 'helping people get better' or 'assisting the doctor' are not adequate foundations. The need is for a professional credo, a nursing raison d'être. It was in response to this need that a series of American nurses began to develop their concepts, or theoretical models, of what nursing should be, the best known in the UK being Virginia Henderson. Coupled with this development, there was also a great deal of thought about the methods of planning and documenting nursing care, the process of nursing or nursing process as it has become known.

The first step here, therefore, is to look at models of nursing and to see if there is one of most use in A & E; the second part of the chapter will examine how that model can be used as a foundation for the nursing process in a typical busy unit.

A good place to start in looking for a model of nursing for A & E is with Henderson, as Henderson's model is used as the basis for much curriculum planning in the UK. She postulated that there were 14 basic human needs or requirements (e.g. the need to breathe normally, the need to drink and the need to sleep and rest) and that unfulfilled needs will lead to a loss of the independence which, according to Henderson, all humans strive to attain. It is a logical step from this to define the goal of nursing as the restoration of independence by satisfying unmet patient needs.

In A & E work, nurses are confronted often with a patient who will be going home from the department. This means that he or she will have to be responsible for *self-care* in conjunction with family and others. Patients may be thought of as being on a continuum of dependency: as they recover from their injury or illness, the amount of care that they need performing for them by others will decrease, while the amount of self-care that they can perform will increase. The emphasis on self-care and the continuum of dependency suggests that as a model we want something a little different from Henderson: furthermore, when we move on to making the model work in a nursing process framework, we will see that assessment is a key element, and the 14 needs of Henderson make for a time and paper consuming exercise when assessment is full. Is there an alternative model that contains these key elements and at the same time permits an assessment that is rapid enough for *practical* use in A & E?

The reader is recommended to study the work of Dorothea Orem (1980), as it is her model of nursing that will be considered here in relation to A & E nursing. Briefly, Orem is concerned with the human being's ability to provide for his or her own self-care and she sees nursing as giving assistance so that a person may meet their own self-care requirements. In normal health, humans look after themselves in six areas of activity which Orem calls Universal Self-Care Demands; on the other hand, when humans are ill, they have three areas of Health Deviation Self-Care Demands—these areas are human structure, human functioning and human behaviour. These two types of self-care demands— Universal and Health Deviation—make up the basis for the nursing assessment of the A & E patient.

Orem views nursing as moving from a wholly compensatory phase when the patient has no active role in meeting self-care demands, through to a partly compensatory phase, and on to a final educational-developmental stage where the nurse is providing advice and teaching to allow the patient to achieve full self-care. This view is very appropriate for A & E, as is Orem's inclusion of the family and significant others in assisting the patient to meet self care-demands, given that the destination of most A & E patients is home.

Orem encourages nurses to anticipate potential problems and to include the family circumstances in care planning, and most important of all, she induces nurses to think about how the patient will manage *on their own at home* (or on the ward if they are to be admitted). Orem's model promotes the idea of nursing care in parallel to the normal process of recovery and rehabilitation from injury as the patient moves along the continuum of dependency. It gives a concise and relevant assessment model from which can be derived a care plan that will help nurses to avoid the sort of pitfalls that are all too familiar in A & E—such as when the patient returns a few days later with their plaster of Paris or dressings in disarray, or when they fail to keep their appointment or to take their medication (e.g. antibiotics), or when they are brought back by the family as 'just unable to cope'. The common denominator for these sort of care failures is that the patient could not practice adequate self-care because either they were not given the information that was necessary in a way they could understand, or because the self-care targets that were set were unrealistic.

Orem's model will be used throughout the book in the hope that it will be possible to show how to avoid these sorts of self-care problems, and at the same time to have a sound theoretical basis for the process of nursing in A & E.

The Nursing Process in A & E

The rationale behind the nursing process is the provision of individua- lised care tailored to suit the needs of each individual patient, carried out in a logical, problem-solving way and properly documented. The pro- cess commences with assessment of the patient's problems, after which goals are set for the *patient* to achieve. Care is planned around these goals and implemented, and the success or failure of the care plan in achieving patient goals is then evaluated. This can lead to modification of the care plan in the light of its success or otherwise.

Many A & E nurses might argue that the nursing process is all well and good on a ward, where staff have the time to write out all the docu- mentation that has become associated with the nursing process, especially when used in conjunction with Henderson's model of nursing and its 14 basic needs. When dealing with 20 patients a day, there is time to plan individualised patient care. But what about the 200 patients seen in a day by a typically busy A & E unit? Surely it is not practical to write care plans for all those people? It is very difficult to argue with this prob- lem when it is couched in terms of the numbers of patients seen per day. Paradoxically, however, this large number of patients means precisely that A & E nurses *do* need a logical, organised and problem-solving approach to nursing.

How then can patients be treated as individuals, with care tailored to suit their needs, and at the same time, how can nurses plan care to avoid the problems arising from the communication failure, the oversights and the pressure of work that come from handling such large numbers of people?

There are two approaches to the problem, both of which involve using the nursing process, but in different ways. First, it should be noted that the nursing process does not necessarily involve the writing down of large quantities of information and the filling-in of forms. It was never intended to be a bureaucratic chore, which unfortunately in some areas it has become, but rather a way of thinking about how to organise nursing care. In other words, for many patients, documentation is not necessary; the nursing process is in the nurse's head and for many of the minor cases seen in A & E, the nurse only needs to *think* the nursing process in order to carry out logical, problem-solving, individualised nursing care.

A typical example will illustrate the point. A young woman with a painful swollen ankle is diagnosed by the doctor as not having broken any bones, but she still has to get home and is in need of some pain relief. A quick assessment should reveal that she is walking with a painful limp, and it is 4 miles to home. Setting goals for the patient is the next step, and without recourse to paper, it is obvious that the goals are that the patient will get home and will experience relief of pain. The nurses plan and implement care around these two goals; they decide upon elastoplast strapping, coupled with advice about rest and elevation to relieve pain, and offer the patient the use of a telephone to ring a friend to come and collect her or to book a taxi.

In setting goals, nurses must set a time limit for meaningful evaluation to occur (possibly, one hour and six hours respectively in this case), and in order for objective evaluation to be possible, the goals must be couched in terms of observable patient behaviour. By defining the nursing care goals in terms of patient behaviour and by setting time limits, evaluation has been made quite easy. For example, if the patient is still sitting in the A & E department two hours later, the part of the care plan concerning transport has failed; while if after being instructed to return if the pain does not ease, the patient returns the following day, then either the instruction about rest and elevation were not properly understood, or something more substantial than an elastoplast strapping was needed, e.g. a plaster of Paris.

This common example shows how it is possible to *think* the nursing process and implement it without the need for documentation. Alternately, the nurses could have noted the doctor's cryptic instruction 'EPS' (elastoplast strapping), strapped up the ankle in the same way that all sprained ankles are strapped up ('We always do it this way, why should she be any different?'), and left the patient limping precariously to the door clutching a shoe in one hand, with no idea of how she is going to get home or what to do about her still painful ankle when she gets there.

Having seen that one way of looking at the nursing process in A & E is to see it as a way of thinking about nursing care rather than a bureaucratic chore—the nursing process is as much in the nurse's head as it is on paper—it now remains to examine one other way of implementing the nursing process in A & E. If we consider the patient with more substantial problems (e.g. burns, chest pain, a fracture), then it is clear that some documentation of care is needed, together with a formalised care plan. The time involved in writing out an individual care plan in each such case in a busy A & E unit is probably prohibitive. However, it is possible to recognise many similarities in the care requirements of groups of patients with the same complaint such as a burn or chest pain. This has led to the idea of *standardised care plans*, drawn up in advance and based on the common elements that are expected to be found in the care of each complaint. Patient assessment therefore consists of an assessment that is standardised according to the model of nursing that is being used, while the care plan to be implemented is selected according to the findings of the assessment and from a series of care plans drawn up in advance to cover the main complaints expected in the department. One essential ingredient for the standardised plan, however, is room to 'individualise' it according to specific patient problems.

The Registered Nurses Association of British Colombia has drawn up a series of such care plans (1977), and note that the time saved by having standard plans ready in advance permits more time to be spent dealing with individual problems in each patient's case. Documentation is reduced to a minimum as the care plan is drafted ready for use before the patient arrives in the department; assessment is reliably carried out by following the assessment guide in the care plan, while for new staff and students in particular there is the provision of a framework of care for each patient which can be adapted to suit individual problems as care proceeds. The documentation that is involved serves as a valuable bridge between A & E and either the ward or community services, thereby improving communications. Finally, with standardised plans based on Orem's model of nursing, nurses have a plan ready for use with every patient that requires little actual writing and that is most relevant to the needs of the A & E patient faced with the realities of self-care.

In order to understand standard care plans better, some of the terms involved need definition.

General Nursing Assessment—This is an assessment carried out on all patients where a standard care plan is to be used. The general assessment allows the recognition of immediate problems and allows the patient to be assigned to one of the standard groups (e.g. burn) as well as permitting the identification of individual problems peculiar to the patient that will need incorporation into the standard care plan. (See Figs. 3.1, 3.2, 3.3, 3.4.)

Specific Nursing Assessment—In this second phase of the assessment process, an assessment relevant to the patient's major complaint (as established above) is carried out. The detail of the assessment is standardised in advance for each complaint.

General Nursing Interventions—Interventions carried out in response to the problems identified in the General Nursing Assessment.

Specific Nursing Interventions—Interventions relevant to the patient's major complaint, standardised in advance.

Individualised Nursing Interventions— Interventions around individual problems identified in the General Nursing Assessment which are essential for individual care.

The General and Specific Nursing Interventions and Assessments are all drawn up in advance (standardised) thereby saving time and providing the nurse with safe guidelines for immediate action. The time thus saved is available for individualising the care plan by taking into account individual problems. The sequence in which these steps are carried out will vary with the patient's needs, but a typical sequence is shown in Fig. 3.5

From Fig. 3.5 (p. 41) it can be seen that the nursing process as used with standardised care plans starts with assessment and continues in a dynamic fashion rotating like a wheel around the hub of evaluation. The feedback between evaluation and intervention may be thought of as the spokes of the wheel, and just as without spokes, there can be no wheel, without feedback from evaluation, there can be no meaningful process of nursing. Evaluation is also linked to assessment in Fig. 3.5 because reassessment is an integral part of evaluation, thereby completing the model of the wheel with its spokes.

Self-care Demand	Ability of patient to fill demand			Reason for Patient being unable to meet demand for self-care.
	Fully Able	Partially Able	Not Able	
Patient can provide for intake of: air water food				
Patient can provide for adequate and controlled excretion of: air urine faeces other e.g. sputum.				
Patient can achieve balance between activity and rest: ambulant use hands/arms sleep normally				
Patient can achieve balance between solitude and socialisation. Is patient able to make adequate social contact at home?				
Patient can prevent hazards to life/safety at home?				
Patient can achieve normalcy in: hygiene clothing mentally home environment.				

NOTE: If parts of Section B are not relevant to the patient's care, do not fill in that part of the assessment.

Fig. 3.1 *Standard Nursing Assessment: Universal Self-care Demands.*

A. Is the patient displaying a health deviancy in any of the following areas?			
Function	Present	Suspected	Not Present
i. Airway Respiratory arrest			
Airway obstruction			
ii. Breathing Paralysis due to spinal trauma			
Difficulty in breathing			
Respiratory depression			
Chest trauma			
iii. Circulation Cardiac arrest			
Shock			
Abnormal pulse rate/rhythm			
Chest pain			
iv. Mental Function Unconscious			
Diminished level of consciousness			
Head/facial trauma			
Unequal pupils			

B. What is the health deviancy relevant to the specific complaint of the patient?

Fig. 3.2   Standard Nursing Assessment: Health Deviancy and Self-care. (1) Human Functioning.

(2) Human Structure			
Code	Structure	Present	Comment
1	Laceration		
2	Deformity		
3	Burn		
4	Swelling		
5	Bruising		
6	Broken skin		
7	Rash		
8	Pressure sore		
9	Amputation		
10	Other, e.g. foreign material		

(3) Human Behaviour. (Underline as appropriate.)

   i)   Vocal: nil/moaning/crying/talking (confused)/talking (orientated) shouting.

   ii)   Non-vocal: still/restless/agitated/very active/walking/running/limping.

   iii) Mood: relaxed/cheerful/quiet/uncommunicative/tense/anxious/aggressive.

(4) History of event and why patient thinks he or she is in A & E unit.

Fig. 3.3 Standard Nursing Assessment: Health Deviancy and Self-care. (2) Human Structure and (3) Human Behaviour.

1. Emergency care

   1.1 Airway — Clear by removal of obstructions (manually, suction).
        Maintain (posture, oral airway, intubation).
        Prevent rotation of head relative to spine.

   1.2 Breathing — Give oxygen.
        Ventilate if needed.

   1.3 Circulation — Cardiac massage.
        Connect to ECG monitor.
        Assist with intravenous infusion.
        Control haemorrhage.
        Record 12-lead ECG.

   1.4 Head Injury — Monitor neurological status.

2. Nil by mouth.

3. Undress patient, check for Medic-Alert bracelet, etc.

4. Commence monitoring of vital signs, fluid intake/output, catheterise.

5. Identify patient, locate old notes if any.

6. Notify next of kin.

7. Offer psychological support for patient/family/significant others.

8. Assist as required with diagnostic tests.

9. Arrange ward and necessary documentation for transfer to ward.

10. If patient is for discharge, arrange follow-up appointment for clinic, community care and transport.

11. Offer teaching and guidance before discharge to patient/family/significant others. Check teaching has been effective. Does patient understand?

Fig. 3.4   Standard Nursing Interventions.

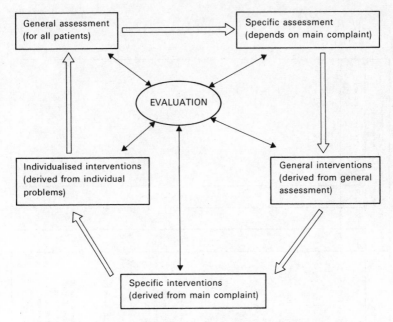

Fig. 3.5 Flow chart to illustrate the use of standard care plans in the process of nursing.

The assessment chart shown in Figs. 3.1, 3.2 and 3.3, based on Orem's model, will act as the general assessment for an A & E standard care plan, while Fig. 3.4 lists the standard general interventions that should be considered for all A & E patients. The specific assessment and interventions will depend upon the nature of the complaint, and some 20 to 30 major complaints may be recognised and planned for in advance in A & E. Figures 3.6a and 3.6b show one such example, burns.

Throughout the book, there will be examples of standard care plans for various complaints as a means of summarising these areas and illustrating the usefulness of standard care planning in A & E.

The nursing process definitely belongs in A & E, and can be implemented either by thinking the nursing process in dealing with minor injuries, or by using standard care plans, based on Orem's model of nursing which, in turn, is more appropriate for A & E than Henderson. This will lead to the minimal amount of nursing time being consumed in paperwork, while providing individualised care within a pre-planned framework.

Date Time	Potential Problem	Patient Goal	Dead-line	Nursing Intervention	Evaluation: Were assessment and intervention carried out as outlined in Nursing Intervention?			
					Yes	No	N/A	Effectiveness in meeting self-care deficit.
				1. Complete Standard Nursing Assessment.				
				2. Obtain data specific to chief complaint: 2.1 Area burnt 2.2 Depth of burn (pin prick). 2.3 Burn agent.				
	Patient is unable to maintain normal respiration.	a. Patient is to clear and maintain patent airway. b. Patient is to take adequate O_2 into lungs.		3. Carry out Standard Nursing Intervention See No. 3 See No. 3				
	Patient feels pain which he cannot relieve.	Patient to achieve relief from pain.		4.1 Assist patient to use Entonox. 4.2 Dress burns with wet soaks (where appropriate). 4.3 Administer analgesic drugs as prescribed. 4.4 Carry out any special treatment for burn agent.				
	Patient is anxious due to pain/fear of disfigurement.	Patient to reduce anxiety levels.		5.1 Offer support to patient and family.				
	Patient's wounds will become infected.	Patient's wounds will not become infected.		6.1 Toilet and debride wound 6.2 Dress wound with Flamazine and non-adherent, aseptic occlusive dressing, maximising function. 6.3 Instruct patient on care of wound/dressing.				

Fig. 3.6   (a) *Standard Care Plan: Burns.*

Date Time	Potential Problem	Patient Goal	Dead-line	Nursing Intervention	Evaluation: Were assessment and intervention carried out as outlined in Nursing Intervention?			
					Yes	No	N/A	Effectiveness in meeting self-care deficit.

Fig. 3.6 (b) Standard Care Plan: Burns—Updating and Individual Patient Problems.

The Extended Role of the Nurse in A & E

As medical theory and practice have advanced over the years, there has been a steady pressure on nursing to keep pace with medicine, and for nurses to be prepared to learn and practice new skills. It was not that long ago, for example, that it was thought that only a doctor could take a blood pressure. In A & E units today nurses are called upon to perform electrocardiography, to suture, to intubate and to administer intravenous drugs, to name but a few 'extended roles'. However, there is no consistency—what is regarded as nursing practice (extended or otherwise) in one hospital may be prohibited in another.

Some argue that nurses should not learn and take on these advanced tasks as by so doing they are only taking on unwanted medical tasks, thereby confirming the nurse in the role of subordinate to the doctor, rather than as an independent professional. It is further argued that the time spent on performing 'extended' tasks is time that could be better spent on nursing care.

On the other side there is the argument that nursing cannot stand still and must move with the times and keep up with progress; furthermore, if nurses do not do certain tasks, who will? The answer could be that there will be a new generation of paramedical technicians, leading to even further fragmentation of care.

The A & E nurse is therefore caught in the cross fire between the two sides of this debate, as are nurses in other specialised areas such as ITU. It seems a little odd, however, to be arguing about the extended role of the nurse when the normal role of the nurse has not been clearly set out. After all if the role of the nurse is not defined, how can talk of 'extended' roles be meaningful?

In order to help the A & E nurse to resolve the dilemmas that occur over the extended role debate, reference should be made to a model of nursing, for it is in the study of Henderson or Orem that the nurse will find a theoretical foundation for what might be considered the role of the nurse. Once the nurse has established a clear philosophy of just what nursing is, in accordance with a theoretical model, then any task that the nurse is asked to undertake can be measured against the yardstick of that model and accepted or rejected on professional, objective groups, rather than—'I would like to do that because it would enhance my prestige' or 'nurses should not do that because they are not doctors and only doctors should do that task'—some of the reasons often heard for and against a nurse taking on a new task.

One example will serve to illustrate the point. Should nurses suture?

According to Orem, a patient with a laceration has a health care deviancy under the heading of body structure, and has a self-care demand as a result, i.e. to close the wound. It is the role of nursing to assist the patient to fulfil their self-care demands; if the most effective way of closing that wound is to suture it, and obviously the patient cannot suture it, then within Orem's concept of nursing it would be a nursing role to help the patient meet their self-care demand by suturing the wound. An objective analysis of a situation, in the light of a model of nursing, leads to a logical answer, without recourse to the difficult debate of extended roles. It is recommended, therefore, that the A & E nurse who encounters problems relating to the 'extended role' consider those problems with the analytical method shown above, always with reference to a model or concept of nursing, and never losing sight of the need for patient-centred care and not task-oriented care. Whatever task is being considered, it should always be possible to integrate it into a total plan of nursing care, otherwise it is not nursing.

The A & E Nurse as a Communicator

How often is a failure in care explained away by statements such as 'nobody told me, so how was I supposed to know'? Communication is an essential ingredient in health care. Reference has already been made to how sociological and psychological factors can impair effective communication with patients and to how, therefore, these factors should be taken into account in planning patient care. Much patient non-compliance is explicable in terms of communication failure, rather than a patient's desire to be 'awkward'.

The development of communication skills is an essential part of nursing and, it could be argued, in no area is communication more important than in A & E. The majority of A & E patients leave A & E to go home, where nurses have no control over subsequent events. The use of an appropriate model of nursing such as Orem's in the delivery of care will help minimise the risk of care failures, but effective communication is also essential if the patient is to understand what is required in terms of self-care after discharge.

A key aspect of communication is the nurse as interpreter of the hospital experience for the patient. For the majority of the general public, the hospital environment is strange and frightening and this is especially true for the elderly and the young. The nurse therefore has a vital role to play in interpreting this experience so that the patient can make sense out of what is being said and done. Patient compliance will tend to increase with patient understanding.

Moving outward from the patient, there are whole networks of communication involving other professional groups and agencies—for example, doctors, social workers, ward staff, the ambulance service and the police— that the A & E nurse will have to communicate with on the patient's behalf. Aids to communication within the unit include the use of a blackboard system whereby each cubicle is numbered and, by having a similarly numbered blackboard plan on the wall which is kept up-dated with each patient's progress, it is possible to keep track of any patient's progress, regardless of how busy the department may be.

An effective way of improving communication with the ambulance service is to send staff out with the ambulance service for experience while at the same time inviting ambulance crews to spend time in the A & E department. Similar exchanges of staff prove successful with community and practice nurses, while the setting up of liaison committees to discuss mutual problems at regular meetings with, for example, the police or psychiatric service, can prove very effective. In short, A & E nurses must realise that they do not work in isolation, but need the effective cooperation of various other groups of staff. It is in the patient's interests if nurses take the initiative in seeking improved communication and understanding with other agencies.

The A & E Nurse and the Law

The police are one agency with whom the A & E nurse will have many dealings, and such is the nature of police interest in some patients that there are going to be occasions when difficult dilemmas of confidentiality arise. On the one hand, it is essential to have a good working relationship with the police, but on the other hand, there is the question of patient confidentiality and police access to information.

If a patient feels that what he or she tells a nurse is genuinely in confidence, and will not be immediately repeated to the police, vital clinical information may be forthcoming that would otherwise be withheld. Examples are in drug use, where it may be essential to know what drugs have been taken, the route and timing of administration, and in wounding cases, where information about the real manner in which the injury was sustained may be withheld, leading to inappropriate treatment and nursing care.

Nursing and medical records have been traditionally held as confidential. This includes the A & E Register, which is a book that on occasion the police may wish to 'browse through'. Such browsing should not be allowed without the consent of the hospital administration. Enquiries about the names and addresses of patients who have attended A & E are best passed on to the hospital administration, although details of patients involved in a road traffic accident (RTA) may be released directly to the police as this is required under law. The police must also be immediately notified of incidents involving firearms and suspected terrorism.

On occasions staff may suspect that a patient has sustained injuries in the act of carrying out a crime which the police are either unware of or are enquiring about. This is a most difficult situation (unless it involves firearms, terrorism or a RTA as mentioned previously) as the demands of patient confidentiality are such that theoretically nothing should be said to the police. However the nurse is also a citizen and, as a citizen, has certain responsibilities before the law. There can be no hard and fast rules and each case must be treated on its merits, but if there is a strong suspicion that an individual has been involved in criminal activity, then a nurse should discuss the case with the doctor responsible for the patient, and a joint approach should be made to a senior administrator (nursing or general) or the consultant in charge.

An example will illustrate the point. A rather scruffy young man comes to A & E with a cut leg. There is a large laceration through the back of his right calf and also through his jeans. The wound is obviously fresh and still bleeding. The friend who is accompanying the patient disappears for coffee while the patient explains his injury in vague terms of 'falling through a hedge'. At this stage the nurse's suspicions are aroused as the wound and story do not match. Enter a policeman and a rather distressed young woman with the story that the woman has just come home to find two men burgling her flat. They broke a window in making their escape, and one of them cut himself in the process. The flat is only a few hundred yards from A & E and the police have followed the blood trail to the front door. Meanwhile a nurse is applying a dressing to the leg, the wound having been sutured. A decision is needed quickly. This real example was dealt with by checking that the woman felt able to identify the men in question, followed by the suggestion that if the police wanted to wait by the main entrance, discreetly out of view, the young woman may be able to identify the men in question in the next few minutes. This was acceptable to the police who easily arrested the two men.

This example shows that by using initiative and commonsense, an awkward situation may be resolved satisfactorily.

Collecting evidence is another area of police work that the A & E nurse will come into contact with. Patient clothing may contain vital evidence and every effort should be made to preserve it. In the resuscitation room, it is often cut off the patient, but if possible this should be done in such a way as to leave undisturbed existing tears or holes as these may give clues as to the weapon used in an assault, for example. Clothing offers clues in 'hit and run' cases as it may contain traces of paint from the offending vehicle, while in shootings there will be gunpowder stains on clothes if the gun is fired from a range of less than three feet. Such evidence is vital to corroborate verbal testimony. Even shoes offer potential evidence for there may be footprints found near the scene of the crime.

All possessions and clothing must, therefore, be safely labelled and stored, for if such evidence is to be admissible in court, it must be possible to establish continuity, otherwise there is the possibility of the evidence being 'planted'. A & E staff will be required to make statements in order to establish continuity of evidence, so the nurse should make mental notes of what is done with clothing and patient possessions during the course of a resuscitation attempt if there is suspicion of foul play.

One problem that commonly occurs involving police is when they want to breathalyse a car driver injured in an accident. As in other cases, they must have the consent of the casualty officer before they can proceed to administer a breathalyser test. If the patient has suffered significant facial trauma, the doctor may refuse consent for a breathalyser if in their opinion the patient's injuries will interfere with the ability to give a full and proper breath sample. However the nurse should be aware that it is not unknown for patients in this situation to offer bribes to A & E staff in an attempt to persuade them to deny the police a breathalyser test. If blood tests are required by the police, a police surgeon will be called to the department to take the necessary samples.

It is essential that there should be a good working relationship between police and A & E nurses, and this relationship may be assisted by trying to see things from the other side's point of view.

Turning away from matters involving the police to more general considerations of legal matters, readers should note that the legal aspects of treating patients against their will are covered in Chapter 16. However, this only refers to the Mental Health Act (1983) and does not cover the rare situation where the patient is a child and the parents' wishes are clearly detrimental to the child's health and welfare. For example, due to their religious convictions, the parents may object to their child being given a blood transfusion and they may withhold consent. It should first be noted that the age of consent for treatment is 16, so whatever the parents may wish for a person aged 16 or over is immaterial—at that age the person is legally able to consent themselves. However, if the child is under 16, parental consent is required before treatment may be legally carried out.

If persuasion has failed to make the parents change their mind, and the situation is serious, the administration and the hospital social work department should be contacted to make an emergency application to obtain a court order to make the child a ward of court. The effect of this order is to remove the child from parental control, usually into the care of a local authority Social Services Department, thereby allowing the necessary treatment to be carried out legally.

The situation may arise, however, where because of serious injuries there may not be time to obtain parental consent or go through the legal protocol and an urgent decision is required immediately. The basic principle that the A & E nurse should adhere to in such situations is to act in what is considered to be the child's best interests while at the same time involving senior hospital management in the case as soon as possible.

Nurses are often concerned about the risk of legal action being taken against them for neglect or malpractice, i.e. being sued for damages. In fact, to date this has never happened, but it is not an unreasonable concern (although it should be noted that part of being a professional is being responsible for your actions). On many counts A & E nurses feel particularly vulnerable to legal action being taken against them, and certainly many general letters of complaint are written about A & E staff to hospitals, which contain a wide range of allegations. Although all the nursing trade unions will support their members, it is strongly recommended here that all A & E staff belong to the Royal College of Nursing in order to obtain the benefit of their professional indemnity insurance cover and also to ensure that if complaints are made at local level, they are well represented by an RCN steward. Such representation is essential if staff are to have a fair hearing.

With regard to the problems of negligence, the legal view is that providing a nurse behaves in such a way as could be *reasonably* expected for a nurse of that position, then whatever the outcome, they are not guilty of negligence. The whole issue hinges on the principle of the nurse's actions being *reasonable*: it is reasonable to expect a qualified nurse to recognise a patient in cardiac arrest, but not reasonable to expect a qualified nurse with no training in the skill to intubate that patient.

The situation can be summarised by saying that, providing the nurse adheres to the twin principles of acting in what is perceived to be the best interests of the patient (adult or child) and only attempting to do things which could be reasonably expected of her or him in the light of their experience and training, then coupled with adherence to health authority policy and membership of the RCN, the nurse should stay out of any serious legal trouble.

Health Education and the A & E Nurse

The National Health Service has been criticised for being a National Ill Health Service, i.e. for emphasising treatment and attempting to cure once a person is ill and for not paying enough attention to the *prevention* of illness.

At present in many parts of the western world, the demand for health care is growing faster than the resources available to meet that demand; the UK is no exception. It is therefore essential to vigorously pursue a policy of prevention in order to try to reduce health demands. It should be noted here, however, that the other side of the coin is campaigning for greater resources to be made available for health care, which means becoming involved in the political process. A dual approach is needed, and nursing as the major caring profession has a responsibility to be in the forefront of both aspects of the campaign for better health.

The A & E nurse is in a very advantageous position to carry out health education. He or she will come in contact with many more members of the general public in a day's work than will most other nurses. Furthermore, the people that A & E nurses are dealing with will tend to be motivated by the fact that they have just had a first hand experience of illness or trauma; they will therefore in most cases be receptive to advice about health or accident prevention.

Simple first aid is one obvious area in which the A & E nurse can carry out health education. Patients often come to A & E with burns covered in butter or toothpaste, with fractured arms where there has been no attempt at splintage, with dressings that are effectively tourniquets that lead to blue hands, or even with tourniquets to control bleeding from simple lacerations. The sight of a patient vomiting the hot sweet tea and brandy that was poured down their throat by a well-intentioned person is still all too common. The nurse has a major responsibility in explaining to the patient about the need to complete a course of anti-tetanus vaccine commenced in A & E, while patients starting a course of antibiotics must have the consequences of not completing the course explained to them. In addition to advice about first aid and medication, there are many other areas where the A & E nurse has a real preventative role, such as in advice about smoking, alcohol and drug problems, contraception, obesity and how to make the best use of Social Services and GPs.

In the future, health care will become increasingly a matter of prevention and the A & E nurse, far from being merely a 'picker-up of pieces', should use the opportunities that present themselves daily to practice health education with patients and their families who, as a result of their own recent experiences, may well be very receptive to advice about health.

References and Further Reading

Bromley B. (1980). Applying Orem's Self Care Theory in Enterostomal Therapy. *American Journal of Nursing*. February. pp. 245–49.

Henderson V. (1969). *Basic Principles of Nursing Care*. Geneva: ICN.

Orem D. (1980). *Nursing Concepts in Practice*. New York: McGraw-Hill.

Registered Nurses Assoc. of British Colombia (1977). *Standard Care Planning in ER*. Vancouver: RNABC.

Riehl J. P., Roy C. (1980). *Conceptual Models for Nursing Practice*. Newark, NJ: Appleton Century Crofts.

Critical Care

Chapter 4

NURSING CARE OF
THE CRITICALLY INJURED PATIENT

The arrival in A & E of a critically injured patient is potentially one of the most difficult situations that can confront an A & E nurse, especially as several patients often arrive together from the same incident. If the nurse in charge does not take a firm, confident grip on the situation at the outset, chaos and confusion can result.

The requirement, therefore, is for a plan of action, known to all members of the A & E team, which will identify and prioritise the major life-threatening problems and the interventions required around these problems. Such a plan involves the well-known ABC checklist of resuscitation—Airway, Breathing and Circulation—and continues with Consciousness (head injury), Spinal injury and Abdominal injury. The seriously injured patient may have problems in one or more of these six areas.

Airway

Pathology

If the patient's airway is obstructed, all other considerations are of secondary importance and immediate intervention to clear the airway for the patient is required. Common causes of obstruction seen in A & E are vomitus, blood, inhaled material such as food or dentures, and soft tissue trauma affecting the neck or respiratory tract. This trauma can be caused by the inhalation of flames or of hot or noxious gases leading to burns of the trachea, by insect stings in the upper respiratory tract, or by a blow to the neck. The unconscious patient will be far less able to protect his or her airway than the patient who is conscious.

Assessment

Airway obstruction is the first step in assessing the A & E patient. Obvious respiratory distress, cyanosis, stridor, the history of the incident and the patient's level of consciousness are all relevant facts in assessing airway patency. The sound of the patient's voice is also important. Is it hoarse? Laryngoscopy should not be performed as it may provoke spasm of the epiglottis or vocal cords. Shining a pen torch into the open mouth is the most appropriate way to examine the upper respiratory tract. Frequency and depth of respirations are important parameters for the nurse to record.

Intervention

The first intervention is to clear the airway for the patient. This can be done manually with the aid of forceps or a gloved hand or with the aid of a wide bore, rigid sucker (e.g. a Yankaur sucker). Dentures often cause obstruction. In the case of an unconscious patient, the airway can be readily cleared by tilting the head back and pulling the chin forward. This action will pull the tongue away from the posterior pharynx. If there is any suspicion of a neck injury, however, this manoeuvre could have disastrous consequences in terms of spinal cord injury. In such a case, a safer procedure is to thrust the jaw forward, but to keep the head in a neutral position.

In serious cases of trauma to the neck region leading to an airway obstruction not amenable to clearance by manual or suction methods (e.g. soft tissue swelling), the A & E nurse may find the medical staff requiring assistance with an emergency tracheotomy, possibly preceded by a needle cricothyrotomy. Needle cricothyrotomy involves making a temporary (and possibly life-saving) entry into the trachea with a large bore (e.g. 14 G) IV cannula attached to a 10 ml syringe which applies a gentle negative pressure. The point of insertion is about 3 cm below the laryngeal prominence (the Adam's apple). After air is observed to fill the syringe, indicating entry into the trachea, the IV cannula can then be connected via an IVI giving set to an oxygen source. Such a procedure can 'buy' the time needed to set up for a tracheotomy. The A & E resuscitation room should have the equipment ready to perform both procedures, and the A & E nurse must know where the equipment is and what is required.

Once the airway is clear, the next intervention is to maintain its patency. The unconscious patient can be turned into the lateral position. Great care, however, is needed if there is any suspicion of a spinal injury and, in such cases, patients are best left flat with other means used to maintain their airway. One simple means of doing this is the oropharyngeal airway which will keep the tongue clear of the airway and which will also allow pharyngeal suction to be readily carried out with a long flexible suction catheter. The airway is introduced 'upside-down' into the mouth and then rotated into the correct position as it is slid over the back of the tongue.

The most satisfactory way of maintaining the airway is probably intubation. In most hospitals, this is a medical task, although ambulance crews are now being trained to intubate in some areas, and with the development of A & E clinical nurse specialists, it may become part of the nurses' role. It certainly fulfils the criteria of what is nursing as discussed in the previous chapter, according to an Orem analysis, in that it fulfils a patient self-care deficit.

At present the A & E nurse must know how to assist with intubation (see Fig. 4.1 for equipment). The first requirement is a muscle relaxant drug, usually suxamethonium, which will be stored in a fridge. The endotracheal tube will often require cutting to length before insertion, so scissors should be kept ready. The laryngoscope blade is then passed on the right side of the midline with the neck extended. The blade is used to elevate the tongue and visualise the glottic opening by pulling forward the jaw at 45° (and not by levering on the front teeth). The tube is introduced into the glottic opening by the right hand. If the tube is too long, there is a danger that it will be introduced into the right bronchus, leaving the left lung unventilated. (The laryngoscope should be checked every morning.) The cuff of the ET tube must be inflated using a 10 ml syringe, and a Spencer Wells clamp is used to ensure the air stays in the cuff. Once inflated, the cuff protects the airway from aspiration, deep bronchial suction is possible and efficient Intermittent Positive Pressure Ventilation (IPPV) may be performed.

As the patient will now be unable to breathe, because of the effects of the muscle relaxant drugs given to permit intubation, the next need is to connect the ET tube to a bag/mask device (e.g. Ambu bag) and an oxygen source via an adaptor and a catheter mount. It is essential that the A & E nurse have the correct equipment to hand immediately, can connect it together promptly and if need be, can take over ventilating the patient. The nurse should not forget the need for tape to tie and secure the ET tube in place.

Evaluation

Evaluation of the patency of the airway after intervention is crucial. The nurse should check the following. Does the patient's colour improve?

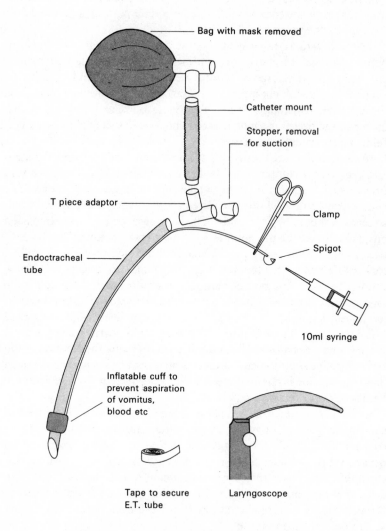

Bag with mask removed

Catheter mount

Stopper, removal for suction

T piece adaptor

Clamp

Spigot

Endoctracheal tube

10ml syringe

Inflatable cuff to prevent aspiration of vomitus, blood etc

Tape to secure E.T. tube

Laryngoscope

Fig. 4.1   Equipment for intubation and IPPV.

What happens to the respiratory rate? Does the chest expand with ventilation in the case of an intubated patient? And is there air entry to both lungs?

Breathing

Pathology

Once the airway is cleared and maintained clear, the next questions are—can the patient breathe normally? And if not, how can the patient be helped to meet this most basic self-care demand? If the patient is making no respiratory effort, the procedure for respiratory arrest must be initiated at once with IPPV. However, the patient may be attempting to breathe but may be suffering from chest trauma which is interfering with normal respiration. If this trauma is serious, it may quickly prove fatal.

A common problem associated with serious chest trauma is pneumothorax in which air gains entry to the potential space of the pleura surrounding a lung. This will lead to the lung's collapse. A pneumothorax can arise spontaneously, without any trauma, due to the rupture of a weakness in the wall of the lung. Tall, slim young males are noted to be prone to this problem of spontaneous pneumothorax (Fig. 4.2A).

The most serious form of pneumothorax is a tension pneumothorax in which the hole into the pleura acts like a one-way flap valve, permitting air entry to the pleural space but prohibiting any escape of air (Fig. 4.2B). The result is a progressive build-up of pressure in the pleural space which will not only collapse the lung on the affected side, but will exert pressure on the uninjured side, leading to mediastinal shift, possible nipping of major blood vessels and collapse of the other lung.

If bleeding occurs into the pleural space, a haemothorax is said to be present. This too will prevent lung expansion, and often occurs in conjunction with a pneumothorax. The quantity of blood involved may be over one litre, so that in addition to serious respiratory impairment, there may also be hypovolaemic shock.

Rib fractures are an extremely painful condition—so painful that proper chest expansion and coughing will be severely restricted, greatly increasing the risk of chest infection. The very serious condition of a flail segment occurs if there are ribs with double fractures, as one segment of the chest wall will no longer be attached to the rest of the chest (Fig. 4.3). As a result, when there is a lowering of intrathoracic pressure (an essential step in respiration) brought about by expansion of the chest

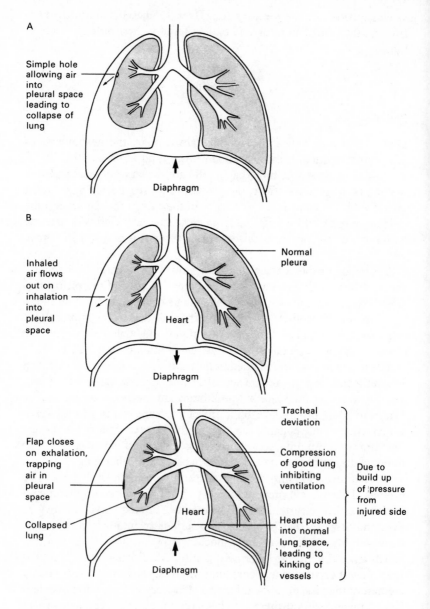

A

Simple hole allowing air into pleural space leading to collapse of lung

Diaphragm

B

Inhaled air flows out on inhalation into pleural space

Normal pleura

Heart

Diaphragm

Flap closes on exhalation, trapping air in pleural space

Collapsed lung

Tracheal deviation

Compression of good lung inhibiting ventilation

Due to build up of pressure from injured side

Heart

Heart pushed into normal lung space, leading to kinking of vessels

Diaphragm

Fig. 4.2   A. Spontaneous pneumothorax. B. Tension pneumothorax.

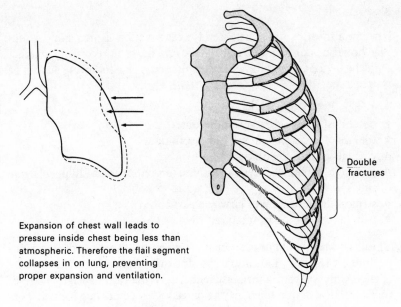

Expansion of chest wall leads to
pressure inside chest being less than
atmospheric. Therefore the flail segment
collapses in on lung, preventing
proper expansion and ventilation.

Double
fractures

Fig. 4.3   Flail segment.

wall, the unattached flail segment collapses inwards under atmospheric
pressure, as the atmospheric pressure will be greater than the pressure
within the thorax. The inward collapse prevents lung expansion. Flail
chest can be readily observed as it results in what are known as paradoxical respirations, i.e. a section of chest wall collapsing inwards when the
rest of the chest is expanding outwards. A flail segment constitutes a
potential life-threatening emergency, especially as it is often associated
with a haemo- or pneumothorax.

Within the lung tissue itself, trauma can cause respiratory impairment in several ways. Major blood vessels may be damaged due to
penetrating injury or severe deceleration stresses. Lung tissue may be
contused, leading to the extravasation of blood into the parenchyma
which in turn will cause anoxia of the tissue. If a high pressure blast
wave passes through the lung, the Spalding effect will produce what
amounts to implosion of the alveolar walls leading to massive damage
and pulmonary oedema which can be rapidly fatal. This effect must be
looked for in all victims of explosions. Finally, there is the possibility of
the inhalation of material deep into the lung tissue. This material can
range from water in drowning victims to noxious gases in burns cases.

Assessment

The chest must be fully visualised for examination. If necessary, clothing should be cut off. The respiratory rate must be recorded, together with the depth and pattern of the respirations. The following should be watched for:

- evidence of cyanosis.
- notably shallow or deep respirations.
- the use of accessory muscles of respiration.
- Cheyne–Stokes breathing.
- gulping, 'air hunger' type breathing (an indication of hypovolaemic shock).
- stridor (an indication of airway obstruction).
- pain (an indication of fractured ribs).

The chest wall should be examined for evidence of trauma, bruising and wounds. Crepitus, indicating rib fractures, may be inadvertently elicited while palpating for bony tenderness (the cardinal sign of a fracture). Surgical emphysema may be perceived as a crackling feeling. This is caused by air escaping into the tissues, typically into the upper part of the chest wall. Paradoxical respirations will usually be apparent if there is a flail segment.

The medical staff's assessment will include the standard percussion and stethoscopic exam, chest x-rays (the area of lung collapse in pneumothorax is seen on an x-ray as a blank area without lung markings separating the lung margin from the chest wall) and arterial blood gases.

Intervention

If the patient is not breathing, IPPV must be commenced at once. Cardiac compression, however, should be withheld until an assessment has been made of cardiac output and the ECG. Using an oropharyngeal airway and a bag/mask connected to an oxygen supply, the A & E nurse should be able to adequately ventilate the patient until arrangements are made for intubation.

If the patient is exhibiting respiratory distress, high concentration oxygen should be applied by mask at a high flow rate. If possible, the sitting-upright position should be adopted to assist respiration. Chest injuries are very painful; the nurse may relieve such pain by the administration of Entonox, which is 50% oxygen and 50% nitrous oxide.

If the patient is conscious, it is likely that he or she will require a great deal of psychological support as difficulty in breathing is a very frightening experience. It is suggested that such a patient should not be left alone at any time, for in addition to the risk of deterioration going unnoticed, it may provoke great fear in the patient.

The need for continual monitoring of respiratory rate and effort cannot be overemphasised as this will give first warning of a deterioration in respiratory function. Cyanosis is a very late sign, and in a significant proportion of the population, i.e. the non-Caucasian population, it is an unlikely sign at all. In non-Caucasians, cyanosis can be seen in the mucous membranes. Drowsiness and confusion are associated with respiratory failure and are due to cerebral hypoxia. In multiple trauma victims, however, it may not be possible to differentiate between when these signs are caused by head injury and when they are due to respiratory failure.

The remaining area of nursing care for respiratory problems concerns supporting medical intervention. In the case of a pneumothorax or haemothorax, the requirement is for a rapidly introduced chest drain, together with an underwater seal, to drain off the air or blood that is

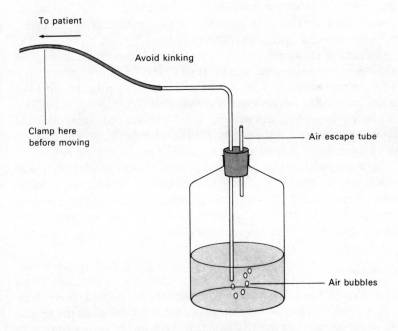

Fig. 4.4   Chest drainage.

compressing the lung (Fig. 4.4). In haemothorax, the drain will be introduced into the 5th intercostal space. In pneumothorax, the drain will be introduced into the 2nd intercostal space. This is because of the simple fact that blood is heavier than air. Most of the equipment for this procedure should be ready in advance in the form of a CSSD pack in the resuscitation room. Great stress should be laid on asepsis during the procedure. Iodine in spirit is usually used as a skin preparation. Local anaesthetic will be administered around the area, followed by a small incision with a scalpel to facilitate the introduction of the chest drain. The nurse should have the bottle ready with a litre of sterile water and should insure that the tubing is connected the correct way, i.e. the drain coming from the patient must be connected to the tube that ends underwater. The chest drain will be sutured in place and the area around it should be dressed with a keyhole dressing secured with elastoplast. If it is correctly inserted, the nurse should observe air or blood draining into the bottle, and the fluid level in the drain will oscillate with the changes in intrathoracic pressure associated with the patient's breathing. The bottle should never be raised above the level of the patient because if this is done, the contents of the bottle will syphon off through the drain into the chest with catastrophic results. If movement of any kind is contemplated, the drain should be securely clamped proximally to its junction with the tube that enters the bottle.

A dramatic improvement in the patient's condition often follows chest drainage, the re-expanded lung being seen on a check x-ray immediately after the procedure. A nurse should accompany the patient during this x-ray, monitoring respiratory status and offering psychological support. If a haemothorax has been present, blood pressure and pulse need close observation because of the danger of hypovolaemic shock. The quantity of blood draining into the bottle needs to be recorded accurately.

In dealing with a large flail segment, the only way to adequately ventilate the lung is by IPPV. This will usually require intubation, although it is worth repeating that the nurse can manage in an emergency with an oropharyngeal airway and a bag/mask until everything required is ready for intubation to proceed in an orderly fashion.

Evaluation

The effectiveness of interventions to improve breathing must be carefully evaluated. Simple mistakes can occur, such as having the oxygen mask connected to an oxygen point that is not turned on or to an empty cylinder. The chest drain can become kinked and can therefore stop functioning, or the chest drain can be connected to the wrong tube so it no longer forms an underwater seal drain.

Patients may be placed in the correct position to help their breathing, but that is no guarantee that they will stay there. They have a tendency to slip down the trolley!

Airway and breathing problems are very dramatic and desperate situations. It is very easy, therefore, for some simple error to occur with potentially fatal results. Continual evaluation must be the rule to be absolutely sure that things are going to plan and that the patient is benefitting from our interventions to assist the self-care demand of normal breathing.

Circulation

Pathology

The next priority in the nursing care of the critically injured person is circulation. Here the principal concern is the possibility of cardiac arrest or of insufficient circulation leading to shock. Therefore, while attention is being paid to the patient's airway and breathing, a nurse should also be assessing the patient's circulation.

The pathology of shock is very complex and there remains much still to be learnt of its nature. However, the main common denominator in all types of shock is reduced cellular perfusion, i.e. when insufficient oxygen reaches the tissues of the body. If this condition is not corrected, it will eventually set in train a series of complex physiological changes which will result in irreversible shock and death. There are three main types of shock—hypovolaemic, cardiogenic and vasogenic—the causes of which are summarised in Table 4.1.

In hypovolaemic shock, the problem is that there is a loss of fluid from the circulation. In cardiogenic shock, there is a failure of the pump, although the blood volume is not affected. While in vasogenic shock, the blood volume is again not affected but rather the arterioles and capillaries dilate, leading to diminished venous return and hence diminished cardiac output, which in turn leads to decreased tissue perfusion, i.e. shock.

The body has compensating mechanisms against shock which come into operation after injury, and which can give rise to misleadingly normal blood pressures in the A & E patient. The main result of these mechanisms is vasoconstriction.

Table 4.1
Classification of shock by cause

Type of Shock	Cause
1. Hypovolaemic	
Haemorrhagic	Blood loss due to soft tissue bleeding, fractures, wounds, etc.
Burns	Loss of plasma in burn exudate.
Dehydration	Major body fluid loss, e.g. due to prolonged vomiting, diarrhoea, or metabolic disorders such as diabetic ketoacidosis.
2. Cardiogenic	Failure of cardiac pump leading to inadequate cardiac output although the blood volume is normal, e.g. after myocardial infarction.
3. Vasogenic	
Septic	Endotoxins from Gram-negative bacteria can cause massive vasodilatation in certain infective conditions.
Anaphalactic	Severe allergic reaction; histamine release increases capillary permeability and leads to dilatation of capillaries and arterioles.
Neurogenic	Loss of sympathetic control leading to dilatation of venules, capillaries and arterioles.

Decreased renal perfusion leads to the release of renin which in turn leads, via the plasma protein angiotensinogen to angiotensin, a powerful vasoconstrictor at the microcirculatory level. In addition, there is adrenaline and noradrenaline release, both of which are vasoconstrictors. This may allow patients to compensate for circulatory loss for some time with a normal blood pressure, especially if they are young and have, therefore, more elastic walls to their blood vessels.

Significant changes will occur in the urine output of the shocked patient. The reduction in circulating volume will reduce glomerular filtration and hence urine formation. Furthermore, the hormone aldosterone and the anti-diuretic hormone will be released as part of the compensatory effect, both of which will diminish urine output. An hourly output of less than 30 ml may be taken as evidence of hypovolaemic shock.

Assessment

In assessing the patient's circulation, we first of all need to know if the heart is beating and if it is, whether it is producing an effective circulation. The A & E nurse needs, therefore, to take the patient's pulse, noting both rate and rhythm. If no radial pulse is palpable, then a femoral pulse should be searched for. Absence of a femoral pulse indicates no effective circulation and cardiopulmonary resuscitation (CPR) should be initiated at once. The patient should be attached to an ECG monitor. If electrical activity appears on the monitor but there is no femoral pulse, the situation should be treated as a cardiac arrest and CPR commenced. The electrical activity will be, in this case, electromechanical dissociation.

If the patient has a cardiac output, the next step is to assess the risk of shock. Continual monitoring of blood pressure is required, and the nurse should bear in mind the possibility of compensated shock as outlined above. Blood pressure should preferably be monitored by the same nurse so that any differences will reflect real differences in blood pressure rather than different hearing abilities or any other subjective factors that can make blood pressure readings unreliable. Respiratory rate and pulse are other key parameters in the development of shock. Both will rise, the respiratory rate in response to the body's need to try to increase tissue oxygenation and the pulse in response to the falling blood pressure. The condition of the skin should be noted as the increased production of adrenaline and the resulting vasoconstriction will lead to a cool, pale and moist skin.

If the patient is conscious or if witnesses are present, a history of the accident is required. The history will often indicate the risk of injuries that may produce hypovolaemia, e.g. trauma to the right upper quadrant of the abdomen will alert the nurse to the risk of liver damage.

The patient's mental state should also be assessed as psychological support is very important.

Intervention

If there is no cardiac output, CPR must be commenced immediately. Management of the airway and IPPV, discussed in earlier sections, are also essential. This section, however, will only focus on how circulation can be maintained (Fig. 4.5).

Effective external compression of the sternum will produce a palpable output at the femoral artery. Research has shown this output to be between one-third and one-half of normal, and a systolic BP of up to 100 mmHg can be generated. The output, however, is thought to be due more to compression of the great vessels in the chest than to compress-

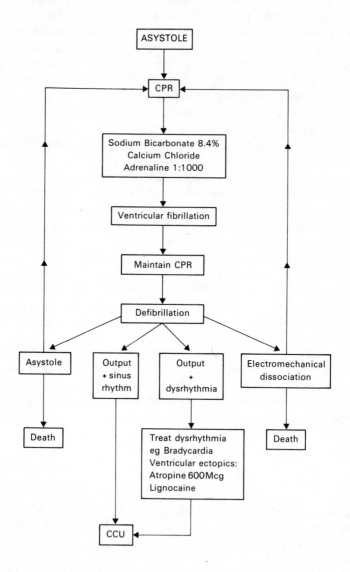

Fig. 4.5   Typical flow chart for cardiac arrest and resuscitation.

ion of the ventricles of the heart. A rate of 60 compressions per minute is recommended with a ratio of 4 compressions to one respiration. Effective external massage is provided by compression of the sternum at a point one-third of the way up from the bottom. Pressure should be applied with both hands, with the heel of one hand having contact with the chest. The nurse's body should rock forward from the hips, thereby applying about half the body weight as the compression force.

It should be noted that recently (and particularly in the USA) it has been argued that, because of the relationship between cardiac output and intrathoracic pressure, *simultaneous* chest compression and ventilation will produce the most efficient cardiac output.

In young children much less force is required—the heel of one hand only for a small child, and two thumbs for a baby. The rate needs to be 80 to 100 compressions per minute, and the ratio needs to be 5 compressions per respiration.

Sternal compression is very dangerous if the patient's heart is beating, therefore a close watch should be kept on the ECG monitor for signs of cardiac activity, and the femoral artery palpated to see if that activity is associated with any output.

The nurse will usually be responsible for drawing up and recording various drugs in a CPR attempt. It will greatly expedite the proceedings if nursing staff know what is likely to be asked for and have the drugs to hand. Table 4.2 is a short list of the most commonly used drugs in CPR.

Budassi and Barber (1984) describe how some of these drugs may be given via an endotracheal tube in a cardiac arrest. Lignocaine, atropine, naloxone and adrenaline are readily absorbed through the lungs, and this route should therefore be considered where an IV line cannot be readily established (e.g. in children). Elam (1977) showed how the onset of action of atropine, adrenaline and lignocaine was 70–80% more rapid in animals in cardiopulmonary arrest when given by an intrapulmonary route compared to intravenously. It should be noted that sodium bicarbonate, calcium chloride and noradrenaline are not suitable for administration via this intrapulmonary route.

Defibrillation is a procedure used if the patient is in ventricular fibrillation and therefore has no cardiac output. The aim of defibrillation is to produce a simultaneous fibrillation of all the myocardial cells. This hopefully will lead to a simultaneous repolarisation which gives the sino-atrial or atrio-ventricular node a chance to resume the pacemaking function.

The nurse needs to know how to charge the defibrillator and to apply either pads or conducting gel to the chest in the correct positions (ster-

Table 4.2
Commonly used drugs in CPR

Drug	Reason For Use
Sodium bicarbonate 8·4%	To correct metabolic acidosis caused by build up of lactic acid in hypoxic tissue. Given from 200 ml polyfusor.
Calcium chloride	Cardiac muscle stimulant, given if there is asystole on the ECG. NB. If it is mixed with sodium bicarbonate, it will form a solid precipitate of calcium bicarbonate and will block the IV route. Normal saline should be flushed through the IV before and after use to prevent blockage.
Adrenaline 1:1000	Cardiac stimulant, given in asystole.
Atropine 600 mcg	Blocks parasympathetic effect on heart; it therefore speeds up a bradycardia.
Lignocaine 50–100 mg	Suppression of multiple ventricular ectopics which may lead to ventricular tachycardia if unchecked. Given by bolus or IVI.
Dopamine	Used to raise BP if profound hypotension occurs after myocardial damage.

num and apex of the heart). If necessary, the nurse should be prepared to defibrillate if the nursing and medical staff have consented to that being part of the nurse's role. The golden rule is to make sure that nobody is touching the trolley or else they too will receive a shock (200 to 400 Joules).

If CPR is successful in re-establishing cardiac output, continual ECG monitoring is required, and further drug therapy may be needed to stabilise the patient's rhythm.

Defibrillation is not used in asystole, the aim there being to produce cardiac activity by use of stimulants such as adrenaline and calcium. The heart may then be defibrillated if appropriate.

The most common cause of shock in the A & E department is hypovolaemia. Immediate nursing interventions should be to elevate the foot of the trolley to try to increase the volume of blood in the vital heart–lung–brain circulation, to administer high concentration oxygen to assist tissue oxygenation, to control any obvious bleeding with pressure dressings and to offer psychological support to the patient.

As hypovolaemic shock is the type of shock most commonly seen in A & E, and as it requires large-scale circulating volume replacement therapy, the nurse must be prepared to offer support to the medical staff in carrying out such potentially life-saving measures. Central venous cannulation will be required as well as a peripheral line, and equipment should also be available for a cut down. Accurate fluid balance charts are required as there may be three drips running at once, together with CVP monitoring. Clear fluids such as normal saline are not satisfactory as they are easily filtered out by the kidneys and can leak from damaged capillaries. Therefore, in resuscitating the hypovolaemic patient, Haemacel is used as a temporary measure until whole blood is grouped and cross-matched. This is an IV solution which has such large molecules that they are not readily filtered out by the kidneys, and due to the osmotic pressure they exert, fluid is moved from the intracellular compartment into the circulation. An IVI warming coil and bath should be available as such is the volume of fluid likely to be given that it may cause hypothermia if not pre-warmed to body temperature. To facilitate the giving of large volumes of fluid in short times, some form of pump is required. A simple device like a sphygmomanometer cuff can be inflated around the IVI bag to force the fluid in quickly.

A supply of O Rhesus negative blood should be available for emergency transfusion if one is needed while the patient's blood is being grouped and cross-matched.

Catheterisation of the patient may be required in order to accurately monitor urine output on an hourly basis.

One form of effective treatment of shock used in the USA is MAST— Military Anti-Shock Trousers—which was developed in the Vietnam War. MAST is a cross between a pair of trousers and a sphygmomanometer cuff inflated with a foot pump. It is an inflatable pair of trousers that has the effect of splinting lower limb fractures, controlling lower limb bleeding, and most important, autotransfusing the patient with a litre or so of ready-warmed, compatible blood, by squeezing it out of the less essential lower limbs into the vital heart–lung–brain circulation. It is only a temporary device and needs very careful deflation, but MAST can bring about a dramatic improvement in a patient's condition in A & E.

Evaluation

Continual monitoring of vital signs is essential to evaluate the progress of the shocked patient. In addition, urine output must be carefully watched as a failure here is a grave sign. The patient's general condition is also a valuable guide to the effectiveness of interventions. Is their skin warmer and less moist? Are they more alert mentally? Repeated checks should be made that the pressure dressing really is controlling bleeding.

Is there another wound that has been missed at the first assessment? These are the sort of thoughts that the nurses looking after the shocked patient should have in order that effective care evaluation may occur.

Head Injury

Pathology

The brain consists of relatively incompressible tissue. Therefore any force applied to it will be immediately transmitted through the tissue. This means that a blow delivered to one side of the head can produce brain injury on the opposite side, as the brain, which is independent of the skull, impinges on the inner surface of the skull.

The skull forms a closed box. The clinical implication of this is that if any bleeding occurs within the skull, raised intracranial pressure will result as there is nowhere for the haematoma to expand, other than to force the brainstem through the tentorial notch or foramen magnum. This condition is known as brainstem herniation.

The majority of head injuries seen in A & E are simple concussions. In concussion, after impacting on the inner surface of the skull, the brain suffers a brief interruption to the reticular activating system. This causes a short period of unconsciousness and amnesia. Bruising or contusion of the brain surface leads to more significant injury and neurological disturbance.

A much more serious injury occurs when a blood vessel is torn, leading to haemorrhage and haematoma formation in either an epidural (between dura and skull) or subdural (below the dura) location, or within the brain itself. The mortality rate for epidural haematoma is 50% and for subdural haematoma 70%, indicating the seriousness of these injuries.

In such major injuries, there is often a short period of unconsciousness after which the patient regains consciousness. During this period of consciousness, the haematoma associated with the bleeding blood vessel develops, leading to a rise in intracranial pressure which will cause a gradual diminishing in the level of consciousness. This period of consciousness is known as the 'lucid interval', and the reason for observation of head injury patients is to try to detect evidence of a diminishing level of consciousness, associated with rising intracranial pressure, as early as is possible so that surgical intervention (burr holes) might relieve the pressure and improve the outcome.

Raised intracranial pressure or haematoma formation may manifest itself by compression of the third cranial nerve (occulo-motor) which controls the iris and hence the size of the pupil. A sluggishly reacting or dilated pupil is evidence of compression of the occulo-motor nerve if it is associated with diminished level of consciousness. There are a variety of other causes of unequal or nonreactive pupils unassociated with head injury. It must be emphasised that this is a late sign that will develop *after* a fall in the level of consciousness.

Skull fracture is not a very reliable guide to the seriousness of the injury, as many patients with a fractured skull have no significant neurological deficit, while other patients sustain serious brain damage without a fracture.

Two types of skull fracture are important, however. Firstly, if the fracture is an open one, there is the risk of infection which may involve the skull itself (osteomyelitis) or the meninges surrounding the brain leading to meningitis. For an open fracture of the skull, there does not need to be a scalp wound as the fracture may be through the base of the skull, communication with the fracture occurring via one of the Eustachian tubes, the mouth or one of the ears. Secondly, if the skull fracture is depressed, the piece of bone pressing on the brain may act as an irritable focus and may cause fitting. A CSF leak may occur due to a tear in the meninges and as a consequence there is the risk of intracranial infection.

Assessment

After assessing airway, breathing and circulation, the next parameter to measure is level of consciousness and changes that occur in that level as this will give the first warning of rising intracranial pressure. It is essential to establish a baseline level of consciousness, and the nearer that baseline is to the time of the accident the better. Witnesses, relatives, ambulance crew and policemen are all key personnel who can help nurses to estimate what the patient's level of consciousness was before arrival in A & E. The importance of level of consciousness as a guide to head injury progress cannot be overemphasised.

Such an assessment must avoid subjective terms like 'semi-conscious' or 'drowsy' which mean different things to different people. The objective Glasgow coma scale is, therefore, recommended. On this scale, consciousness is assessed in terms of motor response, verbal response and minimum stimulus required to produce eye opening. Figure 4.6 shows a coma scale. Alternatively, points can be allocated for each response on

Frequency of Recordings				DATE
				TIME
C O M A S C A L E	Eyes open	Spontaneously		Eyes closed by swelling = C
		To speech		
		To pain		
		None		
	Best verbal response	Orientated		Endotracheal tube or tracheostomy = T
		Confused		
		Inappropriate Words		
		Incomprehensible Sounds		
		None		
	Best motor response	Obey command		Usually record the best arm response
		Localise pain		
		Flexion to pain		
		Extension to pain		
		None		

Fig. 4.6   Coma scale.

the scale starting from zero for no response up to 4 or 5 for the maximum response, the scores for each part of the scale being added together to produce a total.

In assessing motor response to painful stimuli, the nurse is recommended to flex the patient's finger, applying pressure at the proximal end of the proximal phalange with the thumb and pressure with the finger at the distal end of the distal phalange. Note whether the arm is withdrawn towards the patient's body (flexion to pain) or extended away from the body (extension to pain). This latter extensor response indicates brainstem compression, a very serious condition.

Orientation should be assessed in time and space with simple questions such as 'Where are you?' and 'What day is it? and 'What time of day is it roughly?'. Questions such as 'Do you know that you are in the Royal Infirmary and it is Wednesday afternoon?' are not helpful. An answer 'yes' to this type of question is not proof of anything!

In order to determine if the patient lost consciousness, in the absence of witnesses, the nurse should ask the patient to recall the accident. A gap in recall indicates the strong likelihood of unconsciousness, although this period may not be as long as the period of amnesia. Retrograde amnesia refers to a period of amnesia before the accident, while post-traumatic amnesia refers to amnesia after the accident.

In assessing pupil size and response, light of the same intensity should be used in each eye. The nurse should also be checking that when light is shone in one eye, the other responds as well. Unequal pupils in an alert, orientated patient are highly unlikely to indicate any head injury pathology as unequal pupils are a late sign following diminished level of consciousness due to raised intracranial pressure.

Physical signs that should be looked for include scalp wounds. Scalp wounds should alert the A & E team to the possibility of open fractures of the skull and of hypovolaemic shock which can be greatly exacerbated by profusely bleeding scalp wounds, if not primarily caused by such wounds, especially in the elderly. An important sign to look out for is bruising around the eyes (periorbital ecchymosis)—often called 'raccoon eyes'; this indicates an intraorbital fracture or basilar skull fracture. Bruising appearing 12 to 24 hours after injury, behind the ears in the mastoid area, is known as Battle's sign and also indicates basilar skull fracture.

Further evidence of a fracture of the base of the skull is provided by CSF leakage from the nose (rhinorrhoea) or the ear (ottorhoea). Bleeding from within the ear also indicates a fracture of the base of the skull. If there is fluid leaking from the nose, the patient should not be allowed to blow the nose as this could cause contamination of the meninges.

The development of any obvious limb weakness should be reported as this suggests damage to the motor centres in the brain. The nature and duration of any fits must be carefully documented, and medical attention drawn to their presence immediately.

In monitoring the vital signs, respiratory rate is vital, as brain damage may involve the respiratory centre leading to disturbance of both depth and rate of breathing. Respirations may become progressively more shallow and gradually fade away. The temperature regulating centre is thought to be adjacent to the hypothalamus and damage in this region can lead to hyperthermia (temperatures over 40°C). The patient may however be hypothermic as a result of lying still for a period of time after the injury in a cold environment. An accurate baseline temperature is therefore required, taken rectally where appropriate.

A late sign of serious head injury is a rising BP and a slowing pulse. This is explained in terms of the raised intracranial pressure making the heart beat more strongly as blood has to be forced into the brain in order to overcome capilliary resistance. Baroreceptors that are situated in the carotid arteries monitor blood pressure and in response to a rising blood pressure act via the cardiac centre in the brain to slow the heart rate. This is the same mechanism responsible for increasing the heart rate when the blood pressure falls.

Intervention

Airway and breathing must be main priorities in intervention. Administration of high concentration oxygen to head injury patients is beneficial because it reduces cerebral CO_2 levels, and high levels of CO_2 in the brain cause cerebral oedema, thereby raising intracranial pressure further.

In handling and moving head injury patients, the nurse must realise the possibility of spinal injury. Unconscious patients must be assumed to have a spinal injury until proven otherwise, and great care should be taken even if the patient is conscious.

The absolutely vital role of the nurse is the scrupulous monitoring of the level of consciousness, and the maintenance of the patient's airway and respiration.

One final word of caution concerning the nursing management of head injury—many apparently unconscious patients have surprisingly accurate recall of events that occurred and of words that were spoken while they were 'unconscious' in hospital. Perhaps a more accurate description is to say they are 'unresponsive' but possibly aware or 'conscious' of what is said in their presence. Nursing staff should bear this in mind while looking after such patients and talk and behave at all times as if their patient can hear every word they say, because they just might.

Medical interventions that will require nursing support include intubation and ventilation of the patient in order to ensure adequate oxygenation of the brain and airway management, a detailed neurological exam, x-rays, possibly CAT (Computerised Axial Tomography) scanning to accurately define areas of bleeding in the brain (this may be done under general anaesthetic), anticonvulsant or antibiotic therapy as required, and possibly in extreme cases, burr holes which will be drilled in the skull to relieve intracranial pressure and allow clot evacuation. In the past, an osmotic diuretic (e.g. Mannitol) was given to try to shrink the brain by reducing oedema. This required catheterisation. Now, however, this practice has attracted criticism and is less likely to be performed.

The administration of powerful narcotic analgesics in multiply-injured patients is not advisable if there has been head injury, as narcotics have a depressing effect on the level of consciousness. The mistake may be made of assigning a decreased level of consciousness to the effect of the drug, when in fact it is due to rising intracranial pressure. Entonox, a very effective analgesic, may be given by the nurse, however, as its effects last only two minutes. After those two minutes any diminished level of consciousness will be due to head injury and not the effect of the Entonox.

Evaluation

It is essential that senior nursing staff ensure that junior staff understand fully the reasons why they are performing the repeated observations that they are carrying out on the head injury patient. If junior staff do not understand fully, the observations will not be performed accurately and the significance of some vital change will go unreported. Senior staff should monitor the accuracy of their juniors' observations, doing so discreetly and using such a process as a teaching tool.

Spinal Injury

Pathology

The spinal cord is enclosed in a canal extending through the vertebral column with nerves branching off (motor) or entering (sensory) via openings in the vertebrae. The soft nature of the spinal cord makes it very vulnerable to injury with potentially disastrous consequences. A compression of only 2 mm can, for example, lead to the loss of use of a whole limb.

Injury occurs when either a vertebra is fractured and/or spinal ligaments (whose function is to hold the vertebrae in alignment) are ruptured which allows subluxation of the vertebrae. The result will be either compression of the cord or a partial or complete transection. All injuries should be assumed to be unstable until proven otherwise.

The forces causing the injury can be either flexion, extension or rotation, or any combination of these forces. For example, the injury known as a 'whiplash', which is seen in car occupants whose vehicle has been struck from behind, is an extension/flexion injury. Flexion/rotation injuries are seen in accidents in sports such as rugby or gymnastics. These tend to be cervical injuries. The lumbar spine is typically injured in falls where the person lands feet-first and a lumbar vertebra is either crushed or, if there if flexion as well, it is wedged. Alternatively, however, in this case, the vertebra may shatter and produce a burst fracture. The thoracic spine is commonly injured by a direct blow such as a roof collapse in mining or when a person falls, landing on his or her back.

Transection of the cord is tragically an irreversible event. The degree of disability in spinal injury depends upon the amount of damage to the cord and the level the injury is at. Cervical injuries are, therefore, the most devastating, and as cervical vertebrae 3, 4 and 5 contain the phrenic nerve outflow to the diaphragm which is essential for respiration, survival after transection above the level of C5 is very unlikely.

Assessment

Complete transection of the cord produces a flaccid paralysis. It may also lead to spinal shock due to loss of vessel tone (an example of vasogenic shock). Sensation will also be lost. Male patients may display an erection in cord transection. If the injury is incomplete, there will be a mixed picture of sensory/motor loss. The nurse should, therefore, be looking for any weakness or any complaint by the patient of unusual sensations, tingling or numbness. The best way to assess weakness in the upper limbs is to ask the patient to hold the arms out in front of the body for a period of time. If there is any motor weakness, the affected limb will be seen to fall away gradually after a few seconds. To assess lower limb weakness, the patient, lying flat, should be asked to push the nurse away while he or she presses against the soles of the patient's feet with the palms of the hands. Weakness may be perceived in one or both of the limbs.

It is important in the case of neck injury to note how the patient is behaving, as there will be considerable muscle spasm involved in a serious injury. The patient will tend to hold their neck with both hands. Such behaviour in a patient should act as a warning sign of significant injury.

Intervention

All head and multiply injured patients must be assumed to have an unstable spinal injury until proven otherwise. This requires minimal movement of the patient, and then only in a carefully controlled way. In transferring them to the A & E trolley, the ambulance scoop should be used if one is available. Otherwise at least four people must make the lift with a fifth person supporting the head and neck to prevent movement of the cervical spine. The head should be immobilised with sandbags where practical, and a cervical collar applied. The soft foam type are less than 100% effective in immobilising the neck and, therefore, either a rigid splint or a vacuum suction splint should be used.

The patient should be kept flat at all times, turning being accomplished using the log rolling technique. The principle of this is to move the patient in such a way that the spine remains in a straight line and no part of the spine moves relative to another. This will need four people to perform properly. The person in charge of the movement is the person who is bridging the injured part of the spine with their hands. As the patient is being cared for in a flat position, there should be a nurse with the patient at all times, and suction equipment must be immediately available in case of vomiting.

If the patient is conscious and aware of the possibility of spinal injury, the nurse must be prepared for anxious questions from the patient and also from the family. Such questions are very difficult to deal with, but they must be answered honestly and realistically. The patient will need a great deal of psychological support in this sort of situation.

In the A & E department the aim is to prevent any further worsening of the situation by not allowing displacement to occur in a potentially unstable injury. The immediate aim of the medical treatment after a detailed neurological exam and radiography will be to stabilise the spine. This will usually involve traction applied via the skull in the short term. Long-term options include operative fixation or the use of plaster of Paris to make a plaster jacket or a Minerva plaster. The patient may be immobilised in halo traction.

For the spine-injured patient, there will be many long-term problems involving bowel and bladder training, chest and urinary tract infections, pressure sores, rehabilitation, and social and psychological trauma.

Abdominal Trauma

Pathology

The seriously injured patient can have an almost infinite variety of abdominal lesions. They can be due to blunt trauma such as a severe blow, to crushing, or to deceleration forces associated with high velocity road accidents. Alternatively, there can be a penetrating injury due to stabbing, impalement or bullet or shrapnel wounds.

The major life-threatening pathology associated with abdominal injury is hypovolaemia, due to either a leaking major blood vessel or the rupture or laceration of a vascular organ such as the spleen or liver. For example, a correctly restrained car occupant in a high velocity collision may sustain a tear of the aorta due to the deceleration forces involved; a person falling from a ladder or a motorbike may take the brunt of the fall with their abdomen, leading to the rupture of the spleen. Penetrating injuries may lacerate major blood vessels as well as the viscera.

A second major area for concern is peritonitis, caused by the rupture of an organ such as the bowel or gall bladder. It can be either an infective or a chemical peritonitis.

Damage to the diaphragm is a serious problem due to the interference that will occur with respiration, and it should always be considered as a possibility in abdominal trauma.

Assessment

In undressing the patient, the abdomen should be carefully examined for external evidence of trauma such as bruising, wounds or 'tatooing.' The phenomenon of tatooing is found where a very high pressure has been applied to the skin through clothing, resulting in the pattern of clothing being transferred to the skin. Examples are commonly found on the chest and abdomen due to seat belts restraining a patient in a high velocity accident, or in victims of assault who have been kicked or struck with an object such as a billiard cue. The relationship of such external markings to the organs of the abdomen should be considered in assessing possible injury.

Small puncture wounds may conceal very serious damage in cases of stabbing. It is very important to try to obtain an estimate of the depth of the wound and the direction of entry in order to assess the seriousness of the injury. Contrary to common belief, the entry and exit wounds of bullets are both small, even with high velocity bullets, yet they may conceal catastrophic damage, especially in the case of high velocity missiles due to the shock wave and cavitation effects of supersonic projectiles (see p. 141).

Close monitoring of the vital signs is required in order to detect signs of hypovolaemia as early as possible. Abdominal girth may be expected to increase with haemorrhage, although it is likely that signs of hypovolaemic shock will develop before a noticeable increase in abdominal girth. Abdominal girth measurements should be made at the level of the umbilicus, the position marked on the skin, and the reading taken by the same person each time, carefully noting how tight the tape measure was pulled. Readings by different people may vary simply because they each apply different amounts of tension to the tape measure.

The appearance of one or two drops of blood at the external urinary meatus is evidence of rupture of the urethra. Patients who are suspected of having urethral damage should be asked to try to avoid passing urine, while the advice of a urologist is sought. All other patients, however, should be asked to provide a specimen of urine to test for haematurea, which may indicate trauma to the kidney. It is unusual for the bladder to rupture unless it is full, which unfortunately it often is in the case of late night road accidents.

Vaginal bleeding (other than menstrual) indicates that significant gynaecological trauma may be expected.

The detailed examination of the abdomen is the province of the medical staff, however, the A & E nurse should be able to recognise bowel sounds, or their absence which indicates paralytic ileus. Nurses should also be able to recognise the guarding sign associated with peritonitis; the patient holds their abdomen tense, lying flat on the trolley, unwilling to sit or bend at the waist as it is too painful.

The recognition of such signs is essential in the initial nursing assessment if the patient is to be correctly prioritised by the nursing staff.

Intervention

Prompt surgical intervention is required after stabilisation of the patient's circulatory status. Nursing staff will be fully involved in IVI and vital sign monitoring, in ensuring that the patient is kept nil by mouth, and possibly in passing a nasogastric tube. The usual hospital protocols concerning any patient going to theatre must be observed as far as is possible.

If there is an impaling object *in situ*, it is best left there until it can be removed under controlled conditions in theatre while the wound is carefully explored. It is conventional surgical wisdom that the track of any penetrating injury must be fully explored.

All patients who are to undergo surgery need psychological support and explanations of what to expect, both before and after surgery. This applies especially to the patient who is to be operated upon in this kind of emergency situation.

One diagnostic test that may be carried out in A & E and that will require nursing support is peritoneal lavage. The aim of this is to discover if there is blood in the peritoneum, which is a strong indication of the need for laparotomy. The test consists of running a litre of normal saline via a peritoneal dialysis catheter and an ordinary IVI giving set into the patient's peritoneum, allowing it to drain off by syphonage and, most importantly, assessing the colour of the fluid that returns. If there is no trauma, it should be clear. Strict asepsis should be followed, and the skin should be prepared with iodine in spirit. The procedure is carried out under local anaesthetic and the small incision is made with a scalpel.

The blood loss may be so severe in some cases that circulatory resuscitation in A & E is not possible and immediate surgical intervention is needed as a life-saving measure. In such extreme cases, the A & E team should be able to get a patient, if necessary, from the resuscitation room on to the operating table within 5 minutes.

Evaluation

It is essential to evaluate whether the patient understands what is being explained—both explanations about what is happening in A & E and those concerning what will happen in theatre subsequently. Psychological support revolves around patient understanding.

In dealing with hypovolaemia, steps such as elevating the foot of the trolley, IVI administration and MAST application can be evaluated by BP and pulse monitoring.

Abdominal trauma may be very painful, analgesia being withheld until the surgical team are sure of a diagnosis. Once analgesia is given, however, its effectiveness in relieving pain should be evaluated. (See Fig. 4.7 for Standard Care Plan: Multiple Trauma.)

References and Further Reading

Budassi S. A., Barber J. (1984). *Emergency Care*. St. Louis: C.V. Mosby.
Easton K. (1977). *Rescue and Emergency Care*. London: William Heinemann Medical Books.
Elam J.O. (1977). The Intrapulmonary Route for CPR Drugs. In *Advances in Cardiopulmonary Resuscitation*. New York: Springer-Verlag Inc.
Sigmon H. D. (1983). Trauma. *Nursing 83*. January. pp. 33–41.

Date Time	Potential Problem	Patient Goal	Dead-line	Nursing Intervention	Evaluation: Was assessment/intervention carried out as listed in Nursing Intervention?			
					Yes	No	N/A	Effectiveness in meeting self-care deficit.
				1. Complete Standard Nursing Assessment (see).				
	Patient will be unable to maintain clear airway.	Patient will maintain a clear airway.		2.1 Manual removal of obstruction. 2.2 Suction. 2.3 Pull jaw forward, tilt head back. 2.4 Lateral position (spinal injury). 2.5 Nurse present at all times. 2.6 Monitor airway. 2.7 Assist with intubation/ tracheostomy.				
	Patient experiences difficulty breathing.	Patient will breathe freely.		3.1 IPPV with bag/mask. 3.2 Administer high conc. O_2 3.3 Position upright. 3.4 Monitor respirations. 3.5 Psychological support. 3.6 Assist chest drain procedure. 3.7 Entonox.				
	Patient unable to maintain sufficient circulation to support life and avoid shock.	Patient will maintain sufficient circulation to support life and avoid shock.		4.1 Connect to ECG monitor. 4.2 Commence CPR if needed. 4.3 Assist siting IVI and giving IV fluids, chart accurately. 4.4 Elevate foot of trolley (MAST). 4.5 Control external bleeding. 4.6 Administer high conc. O_2 4.7 Catheterise.				
	Patient unable to maintain consciousness.	Patient will not suffer harm as a result of impaired consciousness.		5.1 Intervene as for airway. 5.2 Monitor level of consciousness and other neuro. parameters. 5.3 Administer high conc. O_2 5.4 Prevent self harm, e.g. cot sides.				
	Patient's spinal cord may be damaged.	Patient will protect spinal cord from damage.		6.1 Assume spinal injury. 6.2 Support neck/head in moving. 6.3 Apply cervical splintage. 6.4 Position flat. 6.5 Minimal movement/log roll. 6.6 Request patient lie still, explain. 6.7 Psychological support. 6.8 Entonox.				
	Patient's abdominal organs may be damaged.	See circulation.		7.1 See circulation. 7.2 Prepare for theatre. 7.3 Assist with peritoneal lavage. 7.4 Entonox.				

Fig. 4.7 Standard Care Plan: Multiple Trauma.

Chapter 5

NURSING CARE OF
THE CRITICALLY ILL PATIENT

Care of the Patient
with Chest Pain of Cardiac Origin

Pathology

Ischaemic heart disease (IHD) is the most common serious cause of chest pain seen in A & E departments, accounting for some 150 000 deaths per year in England and Wales. The origins of IHD are thought to be multiple. They are most likely to be the result of a complex inter-play of social, psychological and physical factors, rather than the result of a single physical cause. This makes sense for how else can we explain the fact that for most age groups the death rate from IHD is three times higher in males than females? And how else can we explain why Social Classes IV and V have a death rate that is 20% to 30% above the national average compared to Social Classes I and II who are 40% below the national average? Besides gender and class differences, there are also regional differences. The map in Fig. 5.1 shows a marked variation within the UK of death rates from IHD. All this data suggests that we look to our whole environment and social setting for the causes of IHD.

IHD is a disease of late middle age to old age. The death rate from IHD of men aged 35 is about 15 per 100 000. But this rises to 500 per 100 000 at 55 and to 5000 per 100 000 at age 75 (Silman, 1981).

The majority of deaths from IHD occur soon after the onset of pain. One survey reported that 30.1% of those who died did so within 15 min-utes after the onset of pain, and 56.3% had died by 2 hours after the onset (Rawlins, 1981). (See Figure 5.2.)

It is important to differentiate between angina and a myocardial infarction (MI). If the diseased coronary artery circulation is unable to meet an increased oxygen demand from the myocardium (usually due to exercise), metabolic changes occur in the hypoxic myocardium which produce the classic pain of angina pectoris—a diffuse, retrosternal pain

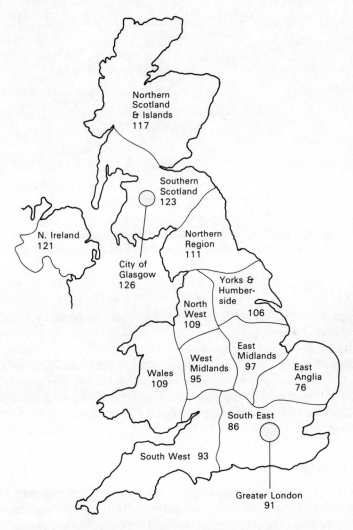

Fig. 5.1   Regional variation in mortality from IHD in men aged 55–64, using standardised mortality ratios (England and Wales = 100). (Sources: OPC, 1979a; Registrar General Scotland, 1978.)

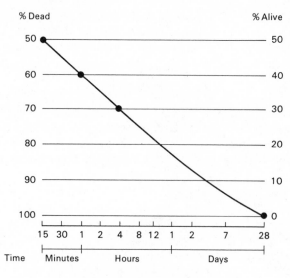

Fig.5.2   Cumulative fatality against time in 348 coronary heart
attacks where death occurred within 28 days (adapted from
Tunstall Pedoe).

which will often diminish with rest. The pain can be easily confused
with that of gastric disorders.

If instead of an inadequate blood supply (angina), there is a complete
occlusion of the blood supply to a portion of the myocardium, that part
will die, and a myocardial infarction will have occurred. The pain is localised in the centre of the chest. It is severe and crushing in nature,
radiates into the left arm and possibly into the jaw, and it is not relieved
by rest.

Assessment

The initial step is to let the patient describe the pain—its intensity, location, duration, what brought it on and whether there is any relevant previous history. The information obtained here should alert the nurse to
the probability of cardiac chest pain and the need to afford the patient a
high priority.

Mental state should be assessed as chest pain is a very frightening experience, and as fear and anxiety can make the condition worse.

Once the general appearance of the patient has been noted—is it consistent with shock?—the vital signs need to be recorded. A rapid respiratory rate is usually seen in cardiac pain. The pulse must be assessed for both rate and rhythm. A bradycardia carries a poor prognosis in acute MI. A systolic BP below 90 mmHg usually indicates shock, and if the patient is indeed suffering from an acute MI, then the presence of cardiogenic shock also indicates a very poor chance of survival. An accurate temperature reading is essential to help to eliminate chest infection as an alternative possible cause of the pain. Research has shown that, for any degree of accuracy in recording temperatures, the thermometer has to be *in situ* for 5 to 8 minutes. A 2 to 3 minute reading will be completely inaccurate.

The next step in assessment is to carry out a 12 lead ECG in order to discover any arrhythmia and evidence of MI or ischaemia. Before performing an ECG, the nurse should explain *in language the patient understands* exactly what is to be done and why—e.g. 'This machine will take a recording of your pulse rate which will help us find out what is causing your pain'. Explanations overheard by the author vary from nothing at all (doctor) to 'This machine will do an electrocardiographic recording of your heart' (medical student) to 'I am just going to do a tracing of your heart' (nurse). The medical student's jargon frightened the patient, while the nurse's language conjured up images of pencils, tracing paper and a procedure akin to brass rubbing. None of the three approaches meant anything to the patient, increasing fear and anxiety as a result.

If nurses are to perform ECGs in A & E, they must understand what they are doing. In brief, they are recording the electrical activity of the heart with a delicate and sensitive machine. The machine should be handled with respect, and every effort should be made to obtain good electrical contact. A conducting medium is required for good contact (e.g. gel). The electrode should not be positioned on hairy parts of the body—the inside of the arms should be used and a razor for removing excess hair should always be on the ECG trolley. Patient movement, muscle tremor, and simple mains electric background hum will all cause interference.

Of the leads that are attached to the limbs, the right leg lead is an earth and plays no active part in the recording. There are, therefore, three limb leads which the machine uses to record the heart's electrical activity in six different combinations. Each of these leads gives a different view of the heart, together with the chest lead which is also used in six different positions. The result is 12 different views of the heart (see Fig. 5.3) which makes it possible to localise the damaged part of the myocardium depending upon which leads show evidence of infarction. If,

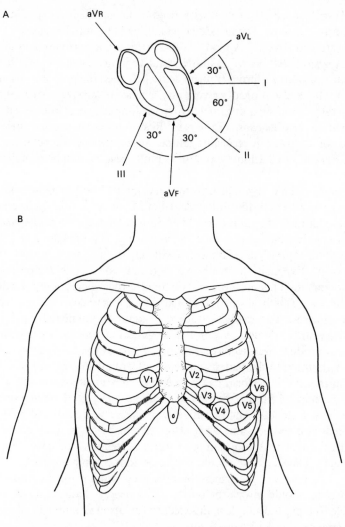

Fig. 5.3   (a) Front view of heart showing how the 6 standard or
limb leads relate in space.
(b) View of chest showing correct position of 6 chest leads.
V1 4th intercostal space, right border sternum.
V2 4th intercostal space, left border sternum.
V3 midway V2 V4.
V4 5th intercostal space, midline of clavicle.
V5 5th intercostal space, tip of clavicle.
V6 5th intercostal space, axilla.
(c) View of heart showing position of V leads.

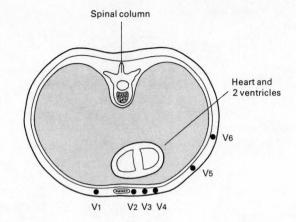

C Spinal column

Heart and 2 ventricles

V6

V5

V1 V2 V3 V4

for example, leads II, III, and aVf show the characteristic changes of an MI, it can be deduced that it is the inferior part of the heart that is damaged.

The basic components of an ECG are the:

P wave	Spread of electrical activity through the atria.
P–Q interval	Conduction of electrical impulse via the bundle of His to the ventricles.
QRS complex	Spread of electrical activity through the ventricles. The Q wave represents the first electrical activity away from the bundle of His in the intraventricular septum.
T wave	Repolarisation of cells ready for next contraction.

Figure 5.4 shows how the heart's conducting mechanism is related to the ECG. The machine is set to record a current towards the electrode as an upwards deflection.

The A & E nurse should be able to recognise the following three ECG changes if correct prioritisation of patients is to occur (see Fig. 5.5).

1. *Pathologic Q wave.* An exaggerated Q wave indicates an area of dead myocardium, i.e. an MI has occurred at some time. However, as this is a permanent change in the ECG, it could relate to an episode that happened a year or more ago. Therefore, on its own, a pathologic Q wave does not indicate an acute MI. Consideration of Fig.5.4 shows that the Q wave is normally lost in the electrical activity of area 2. However if area 2 is dead myocardium, there will be no electrical activity present and the whole of the not normally seen activity in area 1 will be recorded, producing an exaggerated Q wave. The dead area of myocardium acts as an

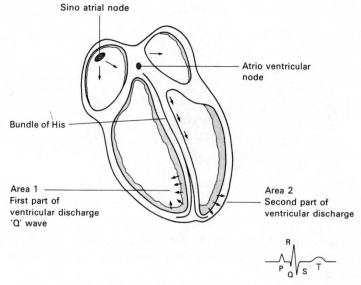

Fig. 5.4   Conducting mechanism of the heart and the ECG.

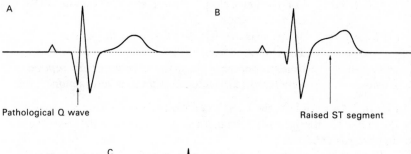

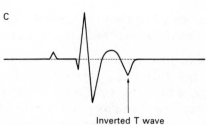

Fig. 5.5   ECG changes associated with IHD.
(a) Dead myocardium: pathological Q wave.
(b) Damaged myocardium: raised ST section.
(c) Ischaemic myocardium: inverted T wave.

'electrical window', allowing us to record activity normally swamped by healthy myocardium.

2. *Elevated ST segment.* This indicates acutely damaged myocardium and may be thought of as being due to the damaged cells leaking potassium ions (K^+) after each contraction. This leads to an excess of positive charges and hence the ST section is elevated above the normal baseline of the ECG (the isoelectric state).

3. *T wave inversion.* This indicates myocardial ischaemia, but not an actual MI.

In addition to evidence of MI, the ECG will reveal if there is any serious arrhythmia present. Therefore, a 30 second rhythm strip from lead II should be obtained, and the patient should be continually attached to a cardiac monitor.

The need for explanation to the patient of what a cardiac monitor is cannot be understated.

The following are the major life-threatening arrhythmias which the nurse should be able to recognise on a monitor (see Fig. 5.6).

1. *Asystole.* No cardiac activity, cardiac arrest. It is essential to check the patient before instituting CPR as disconnected electrodes can produce a trace very similar to that of asystole. Do not defibrillate.

2. *Ventricular fibrillation (VF).* Rapid, quivering of the ventricles associated with a rapid, disorganised pattern of electrical activity. No output produced. Effectively VF is cardiac arrest. It requires defibrillation and full CPR. Check first the patient's condition as electronic gremlins such as loose leads may be responsible!

3. *Ventricular tachycardia (VT).* Caused by a ventricular pacemaker taking over pacing the heart and firing at a very rapid rate, 150–250 beats per minute. There are no P waves, only regular, bizarre ventricular complexes. Cardiac output falls to very low levels. There is insufficient time for the ventricles to fill between each beat. The patient loses consciousness and proceeds to VF unless spontaneous remission occurs.

4. *Ventricular ectopics (VEs).* If there is an irritable focus in one of the ventricles, it may begin firing off pacing impulses itself, leading to premature ventricular contractions or VEs. No P wave is seen, the beat comes early, and the shape of the QRS complex is different from normal as it represents an atypical conduction of electricity through the myocardium. Occasional VEs are not a cause for concern, but if they start to

i) Asystole

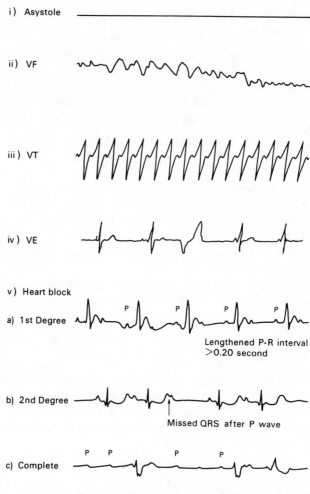

ii) VF

iii) VT

iv) VE

v) Heart block

a) 1st Degree

Lengthened P-R interval
>0.20 second

b) 2nd Degree

Missed QRS after P wave

c) Complete

Fig. 5.6   Serious arrhythmias.

occur in runs, there is the possibility of a VT developing. Bigeminy is the coupling of a normal beat with a VE immediately afterwards. Trigeminy occurs when every third beat is a VE.

5. *Heart block.* First degree block involves a delay in the conduction of the electrical impulse through the AV node. The P–R interval is, therefore, lengthened and if it is greater than 0.2 seconds, first degree block exists. This condition may worsen until some of the impulses are not conducted at all. In this case, P waves may be seen with no QRS com-

plexes to follow and a ventricular beat is dropped as a result. This is second degree block and may progress into a complete heart block (CHB) where the AV node fails to conduct any impulses at all. A ventricular pacemaker may take over to produce a slow rhythm (approximately 20–30 impulses per minute) which bears no linkage to the regular pattern of P waves which may still be seen. Such a slow rate leads to heart failure, and if the ventricular pacemaker fails to fire, the patient collapses with no cardiac output (Stokes–Adams attack) which will be a terminal event unless the ventricular pacemaker picks up again very quickly.

The key steps therefore in assessing the patient with chest pain are to obtain a description of the pain, assess the patient's appearance and mental state, record vital signs, and perform and interpret an ECG.

Intervention

In the case of patients with chest pain, prioritisation of patients for the attention of A & E medical staff is the vital first step in nursing intervention. This is because of the close relationship between the time of death and the onset of symptoms (see p. 84). If the assessment described in the previous section is carried out accurately by the nurse, the patient may be assigned the correct priority.

One of the main thrusts of intervention is to limit the area of damage to the myocardium. To this end, high concentration oxygen should be administered at once. The patient should be cared for sitting upright to assist respiration.

Pain may be effectively relieved by the use of Entonox gas, which has the advantage of being 50% oxygen.

Fear and anxiety must be minimised, partly for humanitarian reasons but also for the good physiological reason that stimulation of the sympathetic nervous system will lead to an increase in the force and rate of contraction of the ventricles, thereby increasing the oxygen demand of already compromised myocardium which can lead to further myocardial damage. The patient should be cared for in a special 'cardiac cubicle' removed from the noise and bustle of the busy department, where monitoring can be carried out unobtrusively, i.e. with the monitor volume control on zero, and with the monitor invisible to the patient (but visible to staff). Explanations of what is happening together with the nurse's own attitude will reduce tension and fear, as will relief of pain, and the presence of family/friends.

The admission procedure to CCU should be expedited as much as possible, remembering the high risk of cardiac arrest in the immediate post-infarction period.

Medical interventions requiring nursing support will be limited to siting and heparinising an IV cannula, and administering powerful narcotic analgesia via that route (e.g. 5–10 mg diamorphine) and an anti-emetic. X-rays should not be obtained in A & E as this delays transfer to CCU; they should be taken later with a portable machine in CCU.

It should be the aim of an A & E unit to be able to transfer a patient with chest pain to CCU within 15–20 minutes of arrival. The transfer should always be undertaken with two porters and a qualified nurse and with necessary resuscitation equipment discreetly placed out of sight underneath the trolley. It is not a good idea to take relatives over to the CCU with the patient in case an emergency should develop in transit. It is better to take them over a few minutes later when the patient has been safely bedded down. It is important to prepare both patient and relatives so that they know what to expect in CCU; the array of monitors and other high-tech equipment can be very frightening and anxiety provoking.

Evaluation

Once a patient has been prioritised, they must not be forgotten. Their progress must be monitored and if necessary they should be afforded a higher priority if their condition changes. Effectiveness of pain relief must be assessed, and in the case of administration of narcotic analgesia, respiratory effort must be closely watched due to the depressant effect of narcotics on respiration. Periodic checks on oxygen administration are required. The patient may remove the mask, especially to answer questions from the doctor, and leave it off.

It is very important to note how the patient's emotional state is progressing, as a modification in the environment (e.g. noise) or in the nursing personnel looking after the patient may be required to reduce anxiety.

Finally the nurse in charge of the patient must be continually checking progress against the target time of 20 minutes for transfer to CCU and not allow things to drift.

Care of the Patient with Respiratory Distress

Pathology

The principle causes of respiratory distress (other than trauma and IHD) are:

1. *Pulmonary oedema*. This in itself is not a disease but rather it is a symptom. The most usual causes are heart failure, MI and other cardiac conditions, but there are many other possible diseases that give rise to pulmonary oedema. The usual picture is one of back pressure from the left side of a diseased heart into the pulmonary circulation. The increased pressure in the pulmonary capillaries interferes with the normal osmotic pressure gradient. This causes fluid to move from the cells into the capillaries. The result is fluid oozing into the alveolar spaces and interfering with oxygen exchange. Normally the amount of fluid in the lungs is equivalent to one-fifth of lung weight. In severe cases of pulmonary oedema, this may rise to the equivalent of ten times lung weight, a twenty-fold increase.

2. *Asthma*. Acute exacerbations may be provoked by many agents such as dust and animal fur. Emotion may also play a major role. Whatever the cause, the result is obstruction of the bronchial tree due to spasm, swelling and secretions which make it very difficult for the patient to breathe out. This leads to the characteristic asthmatic wheeze, hypoxia and severe anxiety. Failure to respond to treatment leads to the severe condition of status asthmaticus.

3. *Acute on chronic bronchitis*. Chronic bronchitis is very strongly class-linked and in winter acute infections in already chronically diseased lungs lead to a very serious illness. The patient is often elderly.

4. *Spontaneous pneumothorax*. See p. 59.

5. *Pulmonary embolism (PE)*. This occurs when a portion of thrombus in a systemic vein or the right side of the heart is dislodged into the circulation and lodges in either the main pulmonary artery (usually fatal) or a smaller artery. When a smaller artery is involved, a PE usually leads to an area of infarcted lung.

6. *Foreign body*. Small children are prone to inhaling all sorts of objects, some of which may lodge in the lower bronchial tree and cause serious chemical damage to lung tissue (e.g. a peanut) and/or areas of lung to collapse distally. Adults tend to come to A & E complaining of animal

bones (e.g. fish or chicken bones) or other food being 'stuck in my throat'. Often they have swallowed the offending object but it has left a tear on the pharynx wall which produces a sensation of an object being stuck.

7. *Smoke inhalation*. Modern synthetic materials contain substances which, when burnt, release toxic fumes. This means that in addition to possible burn injury, the patient may suffer serious respiratory impairment due to chemical lung damage or asphyxia from increased levels of carboxyhaemoglobin caused by carbon monoxide inhalation. (See Table 5.1.)

Table 5.1
Toxic products of combustion

Material	Use	Major toxic chemical products of combustion
Polyvinyl chloride	Wall and floor covering, telephone and cable insulation	Hydrogen chloride (P), phosgene (P), carbon monoxide
Polyurethane foam	Upholstery	Isocyanates (toluene-2,4-diisocyanate) (P), hydrogen cyanide
Lacquered wood veneer, wallpaper	Wall covering	Acetaldehyde (P), formaldehyde (P), oxides of nitrogen (P), acetic acid
Acrylic	Light diffusers	Acrolein (P)
Nylon	Carpet	Hydrogen cyanide, ammonia (P)
Acrilan	Carpet	Hydrogen cyanide, acrolein (P)
Polystyrene	Miscellaneous	Styrene, carbon monoxide

Source: Genovesi, M. G., Tashkin, D. P., Chopra, S., Morgan, M., and McElroy, C.: *Chest*, 71:441, 1977. (P) indicates a pulmonary irritant.

8. *Drowning*. Sea water is a hypertonic solution and therefore it exerts an osmotic pull, drawing fluid into the alveoli. Fresh water, on the other hand, is hypotonic and will readily diffuse into the blood through the alveolar wall. In doing so, however, the contaminants invariably contained in the water will destroy lung surfactant and the fluid will seep back into the alveoli. The result in either case is pulmonary oedema.

Of great significance in immersion injury victims is the time spent in the water and the temperature of the water. Hypothermia develops quickly leading to circulatory collapse. Ironically if the victim is floating in an upright position in the water (e.g. wearing a life jacket), the hydro-static pressure of the water on the lower limbs has a similar effect to MAST, which may preserve life for a considerable period. However, once the victim is rescued, that pressure is lost, the compromised circulation collapses and death occurs within minutes.

Immersion in cold water can produce serious cardiac arrhythmias, including bradycardia which makes the patient appear lifeless upon rescue as there is no immediately palpable pulse or obvious respiratory effort. However, recovery is still possible. This is well documented in cases of persons falling through ice on frozen lakes.

9. *Hysterical hyperventilation.* Hysterical overbreathing disturbs the blood chemistry by blowing off large amounts of CO_2. This leads to an alkalosis and upsets the normal levels of serum calcium. The result is muscle spasm (tetany) which typically causes hyperextension of the fingers and abdominal pain (see Fig. 5.7).

Assessment

The rate and type of respiration should be observed together with the other vital signs. If the patient is mouth breathing, the temperature may be recorded in the axilla for a minimum of 5 minutes. Wheezing indi-

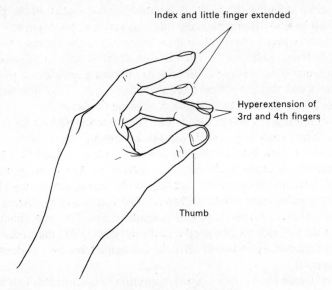

Index and little finger extended

Hyperextension of
3rd and 4th fingers

Thumb

Fig. 5.7 Carpo-pedal spasm.

cates expiratory difficulty and is associated with asthma primarily, but may be found in other conditions, e.g. drowning and smoke inhalation. Stridor indicates difficulty on inspiration, often caused by a foreign body. The nurse should observe whether the breathing is easy or laboured and involving use of the accessory muscles of respiration (the shoulder girdle). A peak flow meter should be available as peak flows form a good guide to progress in treating asthmatic patients.

If the patient is Caucasian, observation of skin colour is a key step in assessment. A cold, clammy pale skin is frequently found in heart failure. Cyanosis, on the other hand, is a late sign and indicates severe respiratory failure. Inhalation of carbon monoxide (CO) produces a deceptively healthy pink skin due to the formation of large amounts of carboxyhaemoglobin.

Mental state must be assessed as respiratory distress is a very frightening experience and psychological support will be essential. Furthermore, confusion is an early sign of respiratory failure as it is due to cerebral hypoxia.

It is important to enquire if the patient has any pain and to obtain a description of it. Central chest pain requires treatment as for a cardiac problem, although it may be a pulmonary embolus that is causing the complaint. More generalised pain over one side of the chest, or extending around to the back, made worse by coughing or deep respiration, and of a sharp stabbing character, is caused by inflammation of the pleura and will be associated with acute infections such as pneumonia.

A history may be very difficult to obtain due to the patient's respiratory distress. Relatives or friends should be closely questioned. In questioning the patient, it is useful to try to phrase questions if possible in such a way that the patient has only to make 'yes' or 'no' answers that can be communicated by nodding or shaking the head.

In examining the rest of the patient, the nurse should look for certain clues. The hands may reveal carpo-pedal spasm, typical of hysterical hyperventilation. Fingers may be nicotine-stained, indicating a heavy smoker who is prone to chronic chest infections. Alternatively, fingers may display the characteristic clubbing at the ends associated with long-standing pulmonary disease. Chronic obstructive airway disease produces a typical barrel-shaped or 'pigeon' chest. The legs should be examined for evidence of a deep vein thrombosis (DVT) that could have led to a pulmonary embolism. Are the calves the same size? Is there calf tenderness?

A specimen should be obtained of anything expectorated. Is it blood stained or purulent?

The medical assessment will include a detailed chest examination, x-rays and arterial blood gasses.

Intervention

The patient should first be sat upright to help breathing and then high concentration oxygen should be administered. The one exception to the use of high concentration oxygen is the patient with a long-standing history of respiratory disease, hence the importance of obtaining a history and checking for signs such as clubbing of the fingers and barrel-chest.

The respiratory drive is normally stimulated by rising levels of CO_2 in the blood. However, in a patient with chronic respiratory disease, the body has adapted to high CO_2 levels and the respiratory drive, therefore, depends upon the secondary mechanism of low O_2 levels in the blood. Giving high concentration oxygen to such a patient will so increase arterial oxygen levels that the respiratory drive will cease to be effective and the patient may lapse into respiratory arrest. Consequently, if assessment indicates the existence of a chronic respiratory disease, oxygen should only be administered in low concentrations—24% or 28%.

The patient who is confused because of cerebral hypoxia may not tolerate an oxygen mask. One solution is to use nasal oxygen cannulae or, as a temporary step, the nurse may hold the mask over the patient's face but without the mask touching the skin.

Psychological support is essential as the patient will be anxious and often very distressed. The nurse's own emotional behaviour will play a large part in determining the patient's (p. 17). Particularly in conditions such as hyperventilation and to a lesser extent asthma, reducing anxiety will help to resolve the respiratory problem itself. The nurse being always visible and providing explanation of what is happening, and why, will help the patient. Nothing could be worse than the acutely distressed patient, abandoned in a dark corridor, awaiting a chest x-ray, alone with the feeling that there is no way they can summon help if they need it. The presence of members of the family may have a beneficial effect on the patient's psychological status, and hence on their breathing. But it can also work the other way, especially when large numbers of people are involved or when certain key individuals are present with whom there is a relationship problem.

Frequent monitoring of vital signs is required, with the respirations deserving maximum attention.

If confusion is present, precautions should be taken to prevent the patient from coming to harm—cot sides, close observation, and reality orientation, carried out at every opportunity, may all be necessary.

Nursing support will be required for medical interventions which usually centre around establishing an IV line and administering drugs via that route. Examples of commonly used drug therapy in A & E for the patient with respiratory distress include IV frusemide 80 mg for pulmonary oedema (diuretic), IV aminophylline 250 mg and hydrocortisone 100 mg for asthma (bronchodilator and anti-inflammatory), IV heparin 5000–10 000 units for a pulmonary embolism (anticoagulant) and nebulised salbutamol 5 mg for asthma (bronchodilator).

In addition to trying to calm the hysterically hyperventilating patient (which often involves the removal of friends), a further useful step is to make the patient breathe in and out of a paper bag. The effect of this is to make them rebreathe their own CO_2 which will increase their CO_2 levels to normal, restore normal blood chemistry, and relieve the muscle spasm (tetany) that exacerbates the distressed state they are in. In many cases, it should be possible to have the patient breathing normally, without tetany, in 5–10 minutes.

Patients in respiratory distress should be afforded a high priority for medical attention. From the nursing point of view, the optimal care will be provided by the administration of the correct oxygen concentration, the positioning of the patient so as to facilitate breathing, the offering of psychological support to relieve anxiety, and continual observation.

Evaluation

Just because the patient is put in the correct position with the correct oxygen mask *in situ* does not mean that they are going to stay that way! They may remove the mask or slip down the trolley. Continual evaluation is essential to pick up these sort of problems and to correct them. Some of the drugs given during respiratory distress are very potent, which makes it essential to closely watch patient progress; for example, aminophylline and salbutamol can have cardiac side effects. To take another example, if the patient has been given IV frusemide, the nurse should note whether they pass urine or not. If not, have they a bladder palpable? Are they in urinary retention as a result?

Due to the significant effect that anxiety can have on respiration, it is important to be continually evaluating the effectiveness of our psychological support for the patient and how the patient is relating to the friends/family that are present.

Care of the Patient with Impaired Consciousness

Pathology

There are many reasons why a person's level of consciousness might be diminished. The following section concentrates on some of the more common causes of patients presenting at A & E with impaired consciousness with the exception of head injury and the effects of drugs and alcohol. Head injury has been dealt with already and drugs and alcohol will be discussed in Chapter 15.

1. *Cerebrovascular accident (CVA)*. The cause may be bleeding from a cerebral blood vessel leading to either a subarachnoid haemorrhage or intracerebral haemorrhage. The onset will be sudden in most cases. Alternatively, there may be occlusion of a blood vessel due to a thrombus (a more gradual onset) or an embolus (a sudden onset).

2. *Fits*. Fits should be thought of as a sign of an underlying disease, such as a brain tumour, rather than as a disease in their own right.

In grand mal epilepsy, the problem is an abnormal discharge of electricity within the brain which first produces a characteristic aura if it is located near one of the sensory centres (e.g. smell, visual disturbance) and then goes on to produce a tonic period of some 30 seconds or so when the patient's musculature goes into spasm and the patient is, as a result, unable to breathe. This is followed by the clonic stage of convulsions which passes into a deep coma from which the patient gradually wakes up. At this stage, often referred to as the 'post-ictal stage', confusion is likely.

3. *Diabetes*. In hyperglycaemic states, the metabolism of fats leads to the formation of ketones whose effects on the brain lead to unconsciousness and brain damage if the ketotic state is not reversed. The body's efforts to excrete the excess glucose in the urine lead to dehydration, hypovolaemic shock and electrolyte imbalance. Ketone formation leads to acidosis which the body seeks to correct by reducing CO_2 levels in the blood (CO_2 dissolves in water to form a weak acid). Hence the deep, sighing respirations characteristic of the hyperglycaemic state.

In hypoglycaemic states, the lack of blood glucose affects the brain to produce drowsiness, confusion and unconsciousness. As urine output has been normal, the patient will not be dehydrated or hypovolaemic.

4. *Acute infections and toxaemic states*. Any acute infection involving the brain, for example, meningitis and encephalitis, will obviously affect the

level of consciousness. Furthermore, any infection that leads to hypoxia (e.g. chest infections) will diminish consciousness as will toxaemic states (e.g. uraemia).

Assessment

The first step must always be to assess airway, breathing and circulation, before moving on to assessing level of consciousness.

A history of the event together with any relevant medical history should be obtained. An epileptic fit may be described or the patient may be known as a diabetic. In undressing the patient, clues such as Medic-Alert bracelets, sugar lumps, out-patient cards and injection sites should be searched for. Identification of the patient is essential, not only so that next of kin can be informed, but also so that hospital notes can be obtained.

In assessing vital signs, the nurse will find further evidence of the cause of the patient's problem. The hyperglycaemic diabetic will be dehydrated and hypovolaemic. The CVA patient will often be hypertensive. Rapid respiratory rate will indicate hypoxia and a pyrexia an infection. The patient may also be hypothermic if they have been in a cold environment for several hours with impaired consciousness. A rectal temperature below 35°C indicates hypothermia.

Blood sugar should always be tested, using one of the modern needle prick stix tests.

Limb weakness should be assessed for evidence of hemiplegia (or monoplegia). Plantar reflexes should be tested by stroking the outer soles of the feet with a sharp object. An abnormal upward curling of the toes indicates an upper motor neurone lesion such as a CVA or a post-epileptic state. Extensor response to pain indicates a brain stem CVA.

A urine specimen should be tested, the hyperglycaemic patient's urine revealing glucose and probably ketones. A uraemic state will cause protein to appear in the urine. An unconscious diabetic patient may be catheterised to obtain a specimen as the presence of ketones in the urine is a very important medical sign.

The medical assessment will include a detailed neurological exam, radiography and blood samples for culture and biochemistry. Lumbar puncture is best performed on the wards and not in the A & E department.

Intervention

The immediate interventions with regard to airway, breathing, circulation and unconsciousness have already been discussed. However, if the patient is conscious but confused, steps must be taken to protect the patient from potential harm. Cot sides should be set up and carefully checked. There should be continual nursing observation and, if necessary, the patient can be nursed on a mattress on the floor. Reality orientation is required with the nurse telling the patient what has happened, what time it is and where the patient is, in order that the patient may make some sense out of the situation. The information should be kept simple as consciousness is impaired.

By providing reality orientation, nurses can help the patient hang on to reality. Try to imagine waking up in totally unfamiliar surroundings, with complete strangers standing around, a gap of maybe several hours in your consciousness and your mental processes impaired by illness. You will then appreciate the importance of reality orientation as a major nursing intervention.

Specific problems revealed by the assessment should be dealt with on their merits. Therefore, if the patient has had a fit, along with care of the patient in a confused post-ictal state, the possibility of the patient having a further fit should be considered. Observation is essential, with the aim of preventing accidental self-harm should a further fit occur. In such a situation, the patient is best left to get on with their fit, intervention being restricted to protecting the head if possible by using a blanket or pillow and by removing any objects that may harm the patient. The nurse should not attempt to restrain the patient or to force an airway into the mouth during either the tonic or clonic stages. This is dangerous and can lead to either the patient's teeth being knocked out or the nurse accidentally being bitten. Once the patient has stopped convulsing, he or she should be turned into the recovery position. The nurse should only then consider the use of an airway and then only if the patient tolerates it. Incontinence may occur due to relaxation of muscle sphincters at this stage. Therefore, the nurse must be prepared to clean the patient accordingly. If fitting is continuous and does not resolve after one attack, status epilepticus is said to be present. This serious condition requires medical intervention to control the fitting (to prevent anoxic brain damage). This intervention usually consists of intravenous diazepam or if needed a general anaesthetic and muscle relaxants.

If assessment reveals that the patient is hypoglycaemic, and if the patient is able to drink, a glucose drink should be given immediately. A supply of Lucozade in the A & E drugs fridge is invaluable. If the patient cannot drink, IV dextrose 50% is given via a butterfly needle; 50 ml is usually sufficient to restore the patient to a normal level of consciousness.

In a hyperglycaemic state, the medical staff will need to correct the dehydration rapidly with an IV infusion. The first litre is usually given as quickly as possible, together with a stat dose of intravenous insulin (one of the rapid-acting varieties). Nursing assistance will be required, together with accurate fluid balance and vital signs monitoring, and usually catheterisation to test for ketones and manage the urine output.

If a pyrexia of over 39°C is present, active steps, such as fanning and tepid sponging, must be taken to reduce the temperature. This is because if it rises to 40°C or above, fitting will often develop.

A space blanket should be used if the rectal temperature is below 35°C.

The possibility of an infection that could be transmitted to other patients in the department should be considered and the appropriate steps taken in line with hospital policy (e.g. disposal of waste and linen).

Pressure area care does not begin on the wards. It begins in A & E, and this fact is particularly important for patients with impaired consciousness. The trolleys in most A & E departments are very hard, and delays in moving patients to the wards are common, therefore patient care should include full pressure area care. Nurses should also check for incontinence which must be cleaned up at once to protect the skin and the patient's own self-image and pride. Nurses should make sure that the patient understands how to summon help if needed for the toilet or any other purpose. The phrase 'basic nursing care' is easily paid lip service to, but this should not be the case in A & E where with the help of Orem's model of nursing we can see that the patient's self-care demands are all met.

Evaluation

Frequent checks should be made of level of consciousness and orientation to assess progress and the effectiveness of reality orientation. Temperature monitoring will reveal the effectiveness of measures such as tepid sponging and the use of a fan. The modern 'stix' tests allow blood sugar to be checked frequently so the effectiveness of care of the patient with a diabetic problem can be evaluated. Regular examination of the patient is needed, to ensure intervention as frequently as required, if there is a risk of incontinence and pressure sores. After a patient has had a fit, it is important to check that the head has been effectively protected; patients can suffer significant head injury from epileptic fits.

Care of the Patient with Abdominal Pain

Pathology

Detailed accounts of abdominal emergencies can be found in many surgical nursing textbooks. It is, however, useful to present a brief table of the most common emergencies seen in A & E (see Table 5.2). Many patients who present with abdominal pain are self-referred or just sent in by a GP without the correct referral procedure to the 'on take' surgical team. The first person they meet is a nurse. Therefore, it is essential that the A & E nurse be able to correctly prioritise such patients.

Assessment

In order to decide upon the priority with which the patient will be seen, the nurse needs to determine the degree of pain the patient is in and the history of the illness and the associated pain. The vital signs are also essential in making this decision.

In assessing the pain felt by the patient, nurses are in a very subjective area, for as already discussed, different people from different backgrounds interpret pain and illness in different ways. It may help to ask the patient to rate the pain on a five point scale, and then try to obtain a description of the pain. Is it constant or intermittent? A steady pain or a gripping sharp pain? Is it localised to one area? Shooting into another part of the body (radiating)? Or generalised over the whole abdomen? Gripping pains of an intermittent nature are known as colic and indicate obstruction of the gut, ureter or bile duct (e.g. biliary or ureteric colic). The pain of appendicitis is localised to the right iliac fossa. The pain of peritonitis is generalised over the whole abdomen.

In taking a history of the illness, the nurse should be checking for vomiting, the type of vomit—whether coffee grounds, fresh blood or bile—and any history of unusual bowel actions, such as diarrhoea, melaena or clay-coloured stools. Previous medical history should be noted as it may contain clues such as changing bowel habits and weight loss (carcinoma?), previous abdominal surgery (adhesions?), and episodes of similar pain relieved by eating (peptic ulceration?). Urine should be tested also.

Table 5.2
Common causes of abdominal pain seen in A & E

System	Disease/Disorder	Typical Age	Comments
1. *Gastro-intestinal*	Indigestion	Young/middle age	Often presents as chest pain
	Alcoholic gastritis	Young/middle age	History of heavy alcohol intake
	Gastroenteritis	Young	Diarrhoea, risk of cross infection
	Constipation	Any	Dietary advice and enema needed
	Appendicitis	Young	Nausea and low grade pyrexia
	Peptic ulcer	Middle/elderly	Haematemesis and melaena. Peritonitis—rigid abdomen; shock if perforated.
	Obstruction	Elderly	Possible cause of obstruction—cancer, adhesions, strangulated hernia. 'Drip and suck'
	Biliary colic	Young/middle age	Colic type of pain
2. *Urinary*	Renal/ureteric colic	Young/middle age	Colic type of pain, haematurea
	Cystitis	Young(female)	Need MSU and urinalysis
	Retention of urine	Elderly(male)	Palpable bladder, catheterise
3. *Vascular*	Aortic aneurysm	Elderly	Hypovolaemia, immediate surgery
	Saddle embolism	Elderly	Circulation to legs lost/impaired
	Mesenteric embolism	Any	Circulation to gut impaired

The nurse should examine the patient's abdomen, palpating to see if it is soft or rigid. The bladder should be felt for. Is it full? An aneurysm will be readily felt as a pulsatile mass in the midline. Stethoscopic examination should be carried out to listen for bowel sounds, their absence indicating a paralytic ileus.

The mental state of the patient, together with any social problems, should be assessed as urgent intervention may be needed. Sudden ill-

Table 5.3
Nursing assessment of abdominal pain—important factors in
prioritisation

Medical Attention is Required

Urgently	Soon	Can Wait
BP less than 80 mmHg systolic	Coffee grounds vomit	BP 110 mmHg or more systolic
Severe constant abdominal pain	Melaena	Soft abdomen
Pulsatile abdominal mass	Palpable bladder	Normal stools
Cold leg(s)	Temperature over 38°C	Constipation
No femoral pulse	Colicky pain	
Rigid abdomen	Haematurea	
No bowel sounds		
Haematemesis		

ness, pain and vomiting constitute a very stressful event for most people. Table. 5.3 is not a rigid set of rules but rather a set of general guidelines. Each patient must be assessed in their own right as an individual.

Intervention

Pain relief is a major priority. This can be achieved with Entonox in many cases. However, analgesia is often withheld by the medical staff at first as the pain is a very important clue in diagnosis. This may need very tactful explanation to distressed relatives. Whatever the patient's pain levels, psychological support for both patient and family is required. The patient should be allowed to assume whatever position is the most comfortable for them.

Surgical intervention is frequently needed. Patients, therefore, should all be kept nil by mouth and, as far as possible, the correct hospital pre-operative procedures with regard to matters such as consent, property and identification bands should be followed. Fear of surgery is to be expected and everything must be done to keep the patient and family informed of what is happening and why. This will help to reduce anxiety.

The traditional 'drip and suck' regime will often be asked for by the surgical team. This requires the passing of a nasogastric tube to aspirate stomach contents and the hydration of the patient by intravenous fluids. Accurate fluid balance together with careful recording of stools is needed.

Evaluation

The degree of relief from pain and anxiety should be noted, further intervention may be needed. Remember that it is the responsibility of the nurse in charge to check that theatre protocols have been correctly carried out by junior staff—for example, is the denture pot labelled with the patient's name? Continual monitoring of vital signs is needed to assess progress. It is important to check that the patient fully understands what has been said with regard to theatre, especially with elderly patients who will often nod in agreement to anything said by doctors without really understanding fully the implications. It is the responsibility of the nurse to check the degree of comprehension by the patient concerning future treatment plans. (See Figs. 5.8 and 5.9, Standard Care Plans: Chest Pain and/or Respiratory Distress, and Impaired Consciousness.)

References

Rawlins D. C. (1981). Study of the Management of Suspected Cardiac Infarction by British Immediate Care Doctors. In *Immediate Prehospital Care* (Basket P., ed.). Chichester: John Wiley and Sons.
Silman A. J. (1981). Routinely Collected Data and IHD in the UK. *Health Trends*, 3: 39–42.
Tunstall Pedoe, H. (1978). The Tower Hamlets Study. *British Heart Journal*, 40: 510.

General Reading

Budassi S. A., Barber J. (1984). *Emergency Care*. St Louis: C. V. Mosby.

See also the journal *Nursing* for many relevant articles, published by Springhouse Corporation, Philadelphia, Pa., USA.

Date Time	Potential Problem	Patient Goal	Dead-line	Nursing Intervention	Evaluation: Were assessment and intervention carried out as in Nursing Intervention?			
					Yes	No	N/A	Effectiveness in meeting self-care deficit.
				1. Complete Standard Nursing Assessment.				
				2. Obtain data specific to chief complaint:				
				2.1 Pain, location, type, what brought pain on, duration, what relieves pain.				
				2.2 Respiratory distress. What brought it on. Duration, type of breathing cyanosis, wheeze or stridor.				
				3. Complete standard nursing intervention.				
	Patient unable to maintain normal respiration.	Patient will have adequate oxygen intake.		4.1 Sit upright. 4.2 Administer O$_2$ (high conc. except for in chronic airways disease). 4.3 Give drugs as prescribed.				
	Chest pain which patient cannot relieve.	Patient experiences relief of pain.		5.1 Give Entonox. 5.2 Give analgesics as prescribed.				
	Patient will suffer stress/anxiety.	Patient will cope with stress, reducing anxiety.		6.1 Psychological support. 6.2 Nursing presence. 6.3 Quiet environment.				

Fig. 5.8   Standard Care Plan: Chest Pain and/or Respiratory Distress.

Date Time	Potential Problem	Patient Goal	Dead-line	Nursing Intervention	Evaluation: Were assessment and intervention carried out as in Nursing Intervention?			
					Yes	No	N/A	Effectiveness in meeting self-care deficit.
				1. Complete Standard Nursing Assessment.				
				2. Obtain data specific to chief complaint: history; blood sugar; urinanalysis; smell breath; test reflexes, limb strength and response to stimuli.				
				3. Complete Standard Nursing Interventions.				
	Patient unable to maintain airway.	Patient is to clear and maintain airway.		4. See No. 3.				
	Patient will suffer injury.	Patient will aviod injury.		5.1 Continual observation. 5.2 Cot sides *in situ.* 5.3 Matress on floor if needed. 5.4 Protect from hard/sharp objects with pillows etc.				
	Patient will fit.	Patient will not suffer harm as a result.		6.1 Intervene as in No. 5. 6.2 Do not interfere with patient. 6.3 Recovery position after fit.				
	Patient blood glucose level too high.	Patient will have normal blood glucose levels.		7.1 Assist with IVI/insulin. 7.2 Catheterise if needed.				
	Patient blood glucose level too low.	Patient will have normal blood glucose levels.		8.1 Give glucose drink. 8.2 Assist with IV glucose.				
	Patient will develop pressure sores.	Patient will have healthy intact skin.		9.1 Turn two hourly. 9.2 Wash if incontinent. 9.3 Expedite transfer to ward.				
	Patient will become (more) confused.	Patient will be orientated.		10.1 Reality orientation. 10.2 Visit by relative/friend.				

Fig. 5.9 Standard Care Plan: Impaired Consciousness.

Nursing Care of the Injured Patient

Chapter 6

FRACTURES AND DISLOCATIONS

Pathology—Causes of Fractures

Fractures are usually thought of as being due to trauma. This is not always the case, however, as repeated stress on a bone can lead to its fracture by a process similar to metal fatigue. Such a fracture is logically known as a stress fracture and is commonly seen in the foot (metatarsal) or the lower limb (fibula). Alternatively, bone can be so weakened by disease that it fails with little or no force involved. This is known as a pathological fracture and is seen, for example, where a tumour has led to secondary deposits in the bone (bony metastases).

Overall, however, the vast majority of fractures *are* due to trauma, and these are described as direct or indirect. In an indirect fracture, the break occurs at some point other than that where the force impacted against the bone; for example, a fall on an outstretched hand may lead to a fracture of the clavicle or wrist. Conversely, a direct fracture occurs when the bone breaks at the point of impact; thus, an over-the-ball-tackle in football leads to a fractured lower third of tibia and fibula.

Types of Fracture

One very important distinction in considering fractures is whether or not the fracture is open or closed. If the fracture site is in direct contact with the outside environment, no matter how small the wound, it is an open fracture. The importance of this consideration stems from the risk of infection which can involve the bone, leading to the very serious condition of osteomyelitis.

Fracture types may be described according to the diagram in Fig. 6.1. Such a classification is important as the orthopaedic surgeon needs to know the mechanism of injury if the fracture is to be successfully reduced. This is because the logical way of reducing a fracture is to reverse the forces involved in the original injury.

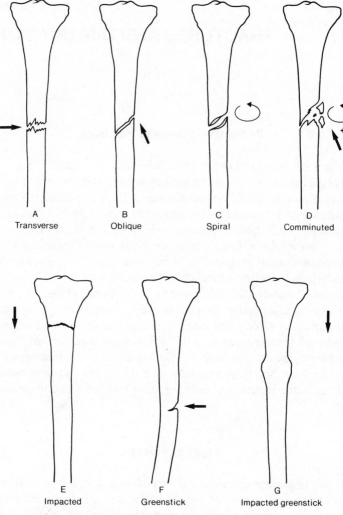

Fig. 6.1 Common patterns of fracture and associated forces.

Fractures and Children

Children's bones have different properties that make fractures a special case when compared to fractures in adults. The much higher proportion of collagen fibres to calcium salts in children's bones means that the bones are less rigid. The result is the greenstick type of fracture where there is only an incomplete break and some cortical continuity remains. As bone growth is occurring at the epiphyseal cartilages located at either end of the bone, fractures involving this region are cause for special concern due to the risk of deformity from damage to the growing area. Such fractures are known as Salter's fractures and are graded I through V in order of seriousness.

Fracture Healing

Fracture healing is a complex process that requires an infection free environment, fracture immobilisation and a good blood supply. Where possible the aim of management is to provide such a situation so that healing can occur conservatively. However, if it is felt that the nature of the fracture is such that this will not occur or that the hazards of lengthy immobilisation are too great (e.g. in the cases of a pathological fracture or a fracture of the femur in an elderly person), then the surgeon may opt to internally fix the fracture by an operation.

The first step in healing is the formation of a haematoma at the fracture site (Fig. 6.2). The haematoma takes little active part in the healing process and is quickly absorbed as cells from the deep surface of the periosteum divide and invade the haematoma. These cells are precursors of the osteoblasts, the cells that play an active part in the construction of new bone. The osteoblasts are responsible initially for the formation of callus which is an immature matrix of collagen and polysaccharides that becomes impregnated with calcium salts and as a result is visible on x-rays. As the callus matures into bone, the final stage of healing occurs with another type of cell, the osteoclasts, helping to remodel the bone by stripping off the surplus bulge from around the fracture site and reopening the medullary canal.

Dislocations

When a join is dislocated, by definition the two joint surfaces are so far displaced that there is no apposition between them. This dislocation also causes serious ligament and joint capsule damage. The term subluxation is used when there has been a partial dislocation so that there is still some apposition of joint surfaces.

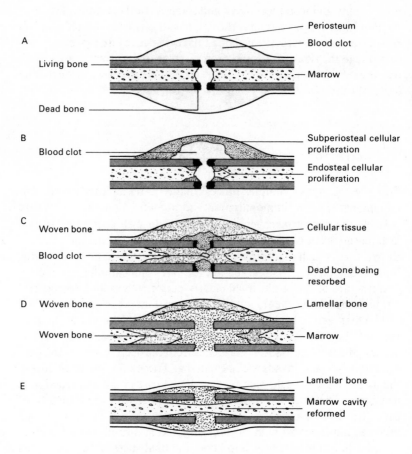

Modified from Crawford Adams J. (1983). Outline of
Fractures, including Joint Injuries, 8th edn. Edinburgh:
Churchill Livingstone.

*Fig. 6.2 Pathology of fractures and the healing of fractures.
(a) Haematoma, with necrosis of the bone next to the fracture.
(b) Subperiosteal and endosteal cell growth. The haematoma is
absorbed. (c) Callus formation. The cells, osteoblasts, lay down
intercellular substance which calcifies to form bone.
(d) Consolidation. Osteoblasts lay down lamellar bone. The
woven bone diminishes. (e) Remodelling. Along the lines of
stress, the bone is strengthened. Elsewhere it is reabsorbed.*

Complications of Fractures and Dislocations

If the fracture is open, the most feared complication is osteomyelitis. Gas gangrene and tetanus are further major complications that are possible with a badly contaminated wound.

If there is pressure on a nerve or blood vessel due to the abnormal position of the bone or to tissue swelling, serious neurovascular complications can arise which in extreme cases can lead to the loss of the limb or to serious disability. Fracture above the humeral condyles can lead to the brachial artery being trapped, cutting off the blood supply to the forearm. This is most often seen in children and leads to Volkmann's ischaemic contracture, a flexion deformity of the hand and wrist. Arterial damage in leg fractures can lead to amputation.

Bleeding from a fractured bone can cause hypovolaemic shock. One litre of blood may be lost from a mid-shaft fracture of the femur and two litres may be lost from fractures of the pelvis. In joint injuries, bleeding into a joint is called a haemarthrosis; such is the limited space within a joint capsule that the result can be a very tense painful joint indeed. If a fracture enters a joint, it is essential for the surgeons to seek as anatomically perfect a reduction as possible as any irregularity left in the joint will lead to the rapid development of osteoarthritis.

Assessment

In assessment, it may be obvious that the patient has sustained a fracture as there is severe deformity and pain. However, many fractures show no obvious deformity—they are undisplaced—and there may be surprisingly little pain, especially in the elderly. Assessment, therefore, needs to progress beyond obtaining a history and beyond just looking at the injured limb.

A cardinal sign to look for is localised bony tenderness, i.e. pain upon palpating the fracture site. This sign is best elicited by gently feeling along the bone and watching the patient for discomfort associated with pressing a discrete area over a bone.

Once the probability of a fracture being present has been assessed, the next step is to assess the amount of pain that the injury is causing the patient and the patient's understanding of the possible injury. Patient compliance with treatment will only be fully forthcoming if the patient understands fully the nature of the injury.

The neurovascular state of the limb should be assessed distal to the injury by feeling for a pulse, the location of which should be marked on the skin. Any wound present should be examined with the possibility of an open fracture borne in mind.

Patient assessment should not be confined to the one limb where there may be an obvious fracture. If there has been sufficient force to break one bone, there may be other less obvious injuries as well, including fractures of other limbs. Vital signs should be recorded to give a baseline from which any deviation indicative of hypovolaemic shock may be detected. The blood loss from fractures alone may cause this condition, in addition to which there is the possible loss of blood from soft tissue injury. As a rule of thumb, an open fracture has twice the blood loss of a closed one.

The psychological and social status of the patient should not be over-looked. This is of great importance in dealing with the elderly because very often it is these factors rather than physical problems that determine management.

Similar considerations apply if the patient has a dislocated joint. Lack of normal joint movement, pain and deformity are the key signs that the nurse will find present upon assessment.

Intervention

Providing that there is no other life-threatening problem immediately identified, the first goal of intervention should be pain relief. Immobilisation of the fracture will make a contribution towards this goal. Home-made or ambulance splints should be removed to allow adequate assessment of the limb (using Entonox as required) and should be replaced with one of two kinds of splint.

If there is a femoral shaft fracture, traction will be required. The traditional method was the use of the Thomas splint with skin traction to overcome the very strong pull of the thigh muscles and to immobilise the fracture. A more modern approach involves the use of the telescopic Tracsplint system developed in the USA.

For fractures of the other long bones, traction is not required in A & E. The best method of immobilisation for these fractures involves the use of a vacuum splint. This is a bag full of polystyrene beads that can be placed around the limb; when evacuated by use of the wall suction, it collapses under atmospheric pressure, forming a rigid splint and moulding to the shape of the limb. Such a system is far superior to old-fashioned methods involving bandaging the injured limb to a rigid splint. In the new system, the limb is not under pressure, the splint is radiotranslucent and the limb is fully visible all the time to allow continual observation of its vascular status. Furthermore, in application, the new vacuum splint is far less painful for the patient.

The next step in relieving pain is to try to minimise swelling by elevation. Hand and wrist fractures should be in a sling; fractures of the lower limb should be elevated by elevating the foot of the trolley. Rings and other constricting jewellery should be removed as soon as possible before swelling becomes a problem.

Movement of the injured limb should be minimised. The situation should not be allowed where successive doctors all want to look at the fracture, resulting in the splint being removed and reapplied several times. Entonox can be freely used for pain relief and in head injury cases this may be essential as the more powerful narcotic analgesics will be withheld for fear of depressing the level of consciousness.

Fear and anxiety will only increase the pain felt by the patient and tend to make for less cooperation. Clear explanation of what is happening and why, together with attention being paid to matters such as informing next of kin, will make a substantial contribution to pain control and the patient's well being.

The pain of a dislocation may be partly relieved by supporting the limb, thereby removing any weight that the joint has to take. Psychological support and Entonox will also be useful for pain relief.

If the injury involves a wound, steps should be taken to wash out any gross contamination with a litre of normal saline immediately. A dressing should be applied, consisting of saline soaks and gauze pads soaked in iodine solution (e.g. Betadine). It may be assumed that the patient will be going to theatre soon, therefore, hospital protocols should be followed as for any patient going to theatre. Formal toilet and debridement in theatre is essential to prevent infection by washing out all traces of contamination and excising all dead or dubious tissue from the wound.

If a fracture is displaced or a joint dislocated, manipulation is required to restore the normal anatomical position of the bones involved. This is frequently undertaken in the A & E department. As nursing assistance will be required, the nurse needs to know something of the procedures which may be carried out.

Gross fracture dislocations of the ankle (the foot rotated at 90° relative to the tibia) require immediate reduction under Entonox by disimpacting the fracture and rotating the foot back to the normal position. If reduction is not immediate, serious neurovascular damage will result. This is a first priority *before* x-ray.

The most commonly manipulated fracture in A & E is the Colles fracture (see p. 124) or other forearm fracture, using the Bier's block tech-

Date Time	Potential Problem	Patient Goal	Dead-line	Nursing Intervention	Evaluation: Were assessment and intervention carried out as in Nursing Intervention?			Effectiveness of intervention in meeting self-care deficit.
					Yes	No	N/A	
				1. Complete Standard Nursing Assessment.				
				2. Obtain data specific to chief complaint: Localised bony tenderness. Deformity. Neurovascular status distal to injury. Presence of wound. Degree of joint movement.				
				3. Complete Standard Nursing Intervention.				
	Patient will feel pain as cannot adequately immobilise limb.	Patient will feel less pain due to limb being immobile.		4. Splintage of limb by: 4.1 Vacsplint. 4.2 Traction (femoral shaft). 4.3 Strap to neighbour (digit). 4.4 Sling (disloc. shoulder). 4.5 POP.				
	Patient will feel pain due to swelling which s/he cannot reduce.	Patient will feel less pain due to swelling being reduced.		5. Elevation of limb by: 5.1 Sling. 5.2 Support on pillows. 5.3 Elevate foot of trolley.				
	Patient unable to maintain normal neurovascular status of limb.	Patient's limb will not suffer impaired neurovascular function.		6. Frequent monitoring of neurovascular status.				
	If wound, Patient's body defences unable to prevent infection.	Patient's wound/bone will not become infected.		7.1 Laverage with NaCl (Sterile). 7.2 NaCl/Betadine dressings. 7.3 IVI antibiotic admin. 7.4 Prepare for theatre.				
	Patient unable to correct bone displacement.	Patient's bones will be restored to correct position.		8.1 Assist manipulation by Dr. 8.2 Prepare for MUA in theatre.				

Fig. 6.3 Standard Care Plan: Fracture or Dislocation of Limb

nique. A double cuff tourniquet is placed around the top of the arm which is then elevated to allow venous drainage before the cuff is pumped up to above arterial pressure as recorded by the attached pressure gauge. Local anaesthetic is then infiltrated into the arm via a butterfly, effectively anaesthetising the whole forearm. The danger is that the anaesthetic drug may leak past the cuff if it deflates. If this occurs before the drug has been bound and rendered inert by plasma proteins, a serious and possibly fatal reaction may occur. For this reason lignocaine and Marcaine are no longer used, the safer prilocaine being preferred. Even with this safer drug, however, the cuff must remain inflated for at least 20 minutes. It is essential that a nurse stay with the patient throughout the manipulation and check x-ray stage, observing the cuff pressure gauge to ensure there is no leak, and observing the patient, who will be probably very grateful for somebody to talk to.

Another common manipulation carried out in A & E is for dislocated shoulders. This technique involves the administration of intravenous diazepam (muscle relaxant) and a narcotic analgesic (e.g. pethidine) before manipulation. The patient is, therefore, not anaesthetised, but will be very drowsy. There is a signficant hazard of respiratory depression so close nursing observation is required in the post-manipulation period.

See summary boxes for brief descriptions of some of the more common fracture and dislocation injuries seen in A & E.

After the fracture has been successfully manipulated (if necessary) and immobilised in plaster of Paris (see Chapter 7), the nurse must consider the problems associated with discharge. These include transportation to home, a follow-up appointment (usually the following day to check the plaster), whether the patient fully understands how to use crutches and/or what precautions need to be taken with the plaster, and finally, whether the patient can cope. In dealing with the elderly, especially those who live alone, it is often the case that the fall that brought about the current injury was the final episode in a steadily deteriorating situation. The A & E nurse must, therefore, carefully assess the patient's ability to cope at home and if there is any doubt, discuss the matter further with the medical staff, in order to fully mobilise community support or explore the possibility of a geriatric admission. The final thought before discharging the patient should be—have they got any analgesia? A timely reminder to the medical staff can save a lot of unnecessary pain with a quick prescription.

If the patient is being admitted because of the fracture, preparation for theatre in accordance with hospital protocols is required. In addition, an intravenous infusion is mandatory for fractures of the femoral shaft to prevent hypovolaemic shock. Fractures of the neck of femur, however, bleed very little and do not require an IVI to prevent hypovolaemia, although one may be erected to ensure adequate hydration of the patient in the pre-operative phase.

Evaluation

The effectiveness of pain relieving intervention should be continually checked, together with the neurovascular status of the limb. Although a limb has been elevated to reduce swelling, it should not be assumed that it will stay that way. Slings can slip and pillows can mysteriously vanish from under legs. Similarly, splinting should be checked at periodic intervals to ensure that it is still functioning effectively.

In evaluating the effectiveness of instruction given to the patient about either plaster of Paris or the use of crutches, it is important that the patient be asked to demonstrate that they have learnt what has been taught. Therefore, the patient should be asked to repeat the plaster instructions to ensure they know what to look for and the patient should be observed walking with crutches. It is not what has been taught that is important, but what has been learnt, and the only way to evaluate patient instruction is to assess what has been learnt.

If the patient is experiencing a minimum amount of pain and anxiety, if their injured limb is safely immobilised, and if its neurovascular status is secure, then the nursing intervention can be evaluated as successful.

Summary Boxes for Common Injuries

Foot Injuries

1. *Fractures or dislocations of toes*
Cause: 'Stubbed toe'. Treatment: Ring block and reduce if needed, strap to neighbouring digit for support with gauze padding. Watch out for swelling.

2. *Metatarsal fractures*
Cause: Heavy weight falls on foot or motorbike RTA. Treatment: Elevate foot, crutches, non-weight bearing (NWB), rest. Watch out for swelling and neurovascular damage.

3. *Fractured calcaneum*
Cause: Fall on to heel. Treatment: Elevate, ice packs, NWB, rest. Watch out for swelling and neurovascular damage.

Lower Leg Injury

1. *Fractured lower tibia/fibula*
Cause: Lateral force. Treatment: If it is displaced, manipulation under anaesthetic (MUA), POP cylinder, NWB will be called for. If a common open fracture, wound debridement will be necessary. If undisplaced, a full-leg, NWB, POP backslab will be necessary. Prone to non-union, usual risks if open.

Ankle Injuries

1. *Fractures of medial and/or lateral malleoli with or without ligament rupture with displacement of talus*
Cause: Rotation and/or abduction or adduction, e.g. twisted foot while falling. Treatment: Simple fracture of malleolus requires a POP backslab, complete NWB for 24 hours, crutches. If ligaments are ruptured, internal fixation with screws will be necessary when swelling permits. Backslab and elevation meanwhile.

2. *Trimalleolar fracture*
Cause: vertical compression, e.g. fall. Joint completely disrupted with posterior part of tibia fractured. Treatment: Internal fixation. Risk of osteoarthritis due to joint surface damage.

3. *Fracture-dislocation of ankle (open)*
Cause: Severe rotational force. Treatment: Immediate reduction under Entonox due to neurovascular compromise. Toilet/debridement, internal fixation. Risk of osteomyelitis, osteoarthritis, gas gangrene.

Wrist Injuries

1. *Fractured scaphoid*
Cause: Fall on to palm of hand, usually in young adult. Treatment: Fracture often does not show on first x-ray, but if there is localised bony tenderness in 'snuff box', treat as fracture with POP to include base of thumb. Untreated, risk of osteroarthritis.

2. *Fractured base of thumb (Bennett's fracture)*
Cause: Longitudinal force, e.g. boxing. Treatment: Involves the joint, therefore, needs perfect reduction (possible internal fixation) to avoid osteoarthritis. POP to include interphalangeal joint.

Forearm Fractures

1. *Fractured distal radius with posterior displacement (Colles fracture, see Fig. 6.4)*
Cause: Fall on outstretched hand, elderly. Displacement requires correction by disimpaction, anterior manipulation and placing hand in ulnar deviation. POP backslab and sling, complete POP applied at 24 hrs.

2. *As above with anterior displacement (Smiths fracture)*
Cause: fall on hand in flexed position. Treatment: Manipulate as above with posterior manipulation. However, a POP which includes the elbow is necessary due to high risk of fracture re-displacing. May need internal fixation.

3. *Fractured mid-shaft radius and ulnar* (see Fig. 6.5)
Cause: High energy injury, often seen in children as a greenstick fracture. Treatment: Manipulation needed under GA for children, then POP. In adults, often internally fixed.

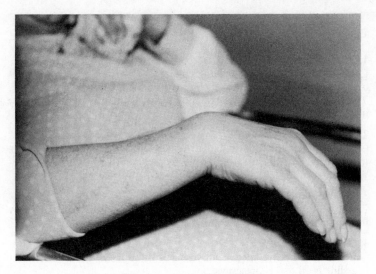

Fig. 6.4   Colles Fracture.

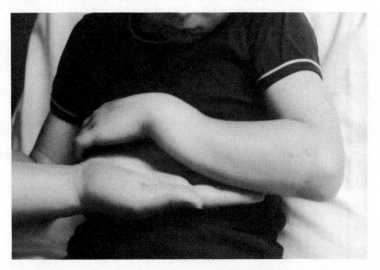

Fig. 6.5   Fracture of radius and ulna in seven year old boy.

Elbow Injuries

1. *Pulled elbow*
Cause: Sudden arm jerk in young child age 2–3. Annular ligament slips over head of radius leading to painful elbow that the child will not move. Treatment: Reduce by pushing forearm upwards and rotating alternatively into supination and pronation.

2. *Dislocation of elbow*
Cause: Heavy fall. Radius and ulnar usually dislocated backwards relative to humerus. Treatment: Needs rapid reduction under GA due to neuro-vascular hazards.

3. *Fracture of olecranon process*
Cause: Fall on point of elbow. Treatment: Either treat by POP, by screw fixation internally or by excision of olecranon process.

4. *Fracture of radial head*
Cause: Fall on outstretched hand, young age group. Treatment: Often rest in a sling is all that is prescribed.

5. *Supracondylar fracture of humerus*
Cause: Fall in childhood. Treatment: Requires immediate reduction under GA due to risk to brachial artery. Long-term risk of deformity due to malunion—'Gun stock deformity'.

Injuries of the Upper Arm

1. *Fractured shaft of humerus*
Cause: Direct violence, usually in adults, or may be pathological. Treatment: Hanging U Slab POP, plus collar and cuff sling, or internal fixation. Complete POP later.

2. *Fractured neck of humerus*
Cause: Fall in the elderly, not usually displaced. Treatment: Sling or collar and cuff; emphasis is on mobility and exercise as the shoulder may become permanently stiff.

Injuries Involving the Shoulder

Dislocated shoulder
Cause: Fall on outstretched hand, usually anterior dislocation. Treatment: Reduce under IV diazepam and pethidine in A & E. Use Kocher method—apply traction along humerus with elbow bent at 90°, rotate arm laterally, carry elbow across body to midline, rotate arm so that hand falls to opposite side of chest. Alternatively pull along humerus with counter traction in axilla.

Fractured clavicle
Cause: Fall on hand. Treatment: Conservative—with sling to support arm. Watch out for pressure on skin from bone ends.

Knee Injuries

1. *Fracture of the tibial plateau*
Cause: Blow from the side rotating femur on to lateral tibial condyle, e.g. car bumper hitting pedestrian. Treatment: After aspiration of haemarthrosis, POP, NWB. Osteoarthritis is long-term problem.

2. *Fracture of patella*
Cause: Direct blow. Treatment: If badly comminuted, patella is excised. If single fracture line, the two halves can be wired together.

3. *Dislocation of patella*
Cause: Flexion of knee. Patella always displaces laterally. The knee is held flexed. Treatment: Easily reduced under Entonox/IV diazepam. POP backslab.

Hand Injuries

1. *Fracture or dislocation of digit*
Cause: Direct blow. Treatment: Strap to neighbouring digit for support with gauze padding between. Encourage mobility. High arm sling for swelling.

2. *Fractured metacarpal*
Cause: Punching, usually fifth metacarpal. Treatment: If angulated, needs reduction and immobilisation in volar slab in Edinburgh position, i.e. fingers extended and wrist cocked back. High arm sling.

Injuries to the Thigh and Hip

1. *Fractured shaft of femur*
Cause: High energy injury in young, pathological in elderly. Treatment: Traction to immobilise. IVI to prevent shock. Theatre for skeletal traction or internal fixation.

2. *Fractured neck of femur (or trochanteric region)*
Cause: Usually in elderly to very elderly a minor fall, or pathological due to osteoporosis. Leg shortened and externally rotated. Treatment: Requires internal fixation within 24 to 48 hours. Major social and psychological problems.

3. *Dislocation of hip*
Cause: High energy injury. Leg shortened and internally rotated. May be driven through acetabulum in central dislocation leading to long term problems with osteoarthritis. Treatment: Reduction under GA in theatre.

4. *Fracture of pelvis*
Cause: In the elderly, usually due to a fall causing fracture of pubic rami; in young people, due to a high energy injury with fracture of pubic ring in two places. Blood loss up to 2 litres. Treatment: IVI urgent, risk of ruptured bladder or torn urethra. In the elderly, should be treated with bed rest. Major injury—requires pelvic sling or external fixation.

Further Reading

Adams J. C. (1983). *Outline of Fractures*, 8th edn. Edinburgh: Churchill Livingstone.

Chapter 7

PLASTER OF PARIS APPLICATION

Basic Principles

The plaster of Paris cast (POP) is an old, tried-and-trusted, effective and relatively cheap method of immobilising a limb. It consists of hemihydrated calcium sulphate which is impregnated into bandage. Immersion in water causes an exothermic reaction to occur—heat is given off—as the hemihydrated calcium sulphate turns to hydrated calcium sulphate which sets to form the hard plaster cast.

There are, however, potential problems connected with plasters. If nurses are to avoid such problems, and to maximise the benefits for the patient, there are certain basic principles that must be observed.

Patient Understanding

The patient must understand what is happening and why. For the best results in applying the POP and in its subsequent aftercare, a high degree of patient compliance and cooperation is required. This is unlikely to be forthcoming unless there is full comprehension by the patient concerning plaster care.

Adequate Padding of the Limb

A POP is very hard both on the inside and on the outside. Therefore, unless it is well padded, there are going to be problems with the skin, and the formation of broken areas leading to pressure sores is likely. There should be a layer of an elasticated tubular bandage (Stockinet) next to the skin, overlaid by one of the proprietary padded bandages that are available for this purpose. Particular attention should be paid to padding bony prominences such as the ulnar styloid and the head of the fibula. The padding should extend above and below the plaster so that it may be turned back over the ends of the POP, preventing skin friction by the plaster edges.

Water Temperature

Water temperature determines setting time: the cooler the water, the longer the plaster takes to set initially. The nurse who is learning the techniques of plastering is, therefore, recommended to always use cold water, remembering to ensure that the bandage has been properly soaked through in the water, with some of the excess gently squeezed out before application.

Movement during Application

If there is any movement of a joint during the application or the initial setting phase, cracks will form within the POP which will seriously weaken the plaster and lead to its failure in the long term. Joints must be held perfectly still during the initial stage of setting.

Moulding

The plaster must be moulded to the shape of the limb in order to maximise comfort and support for the fracture. This means that speed is of the essence in applying the plaster. There must be time before it starts to harden for gentle moulding to be carried out.

Constriction

Tissue swelling accompanies most fractures and ligament injuries. If the limb is encased in a tight plaster, there will be no room for expansion to occur. This will cause compression of the soft tissues in the limb, leading to pain and a significant risk of neurovascular damage.

There are two main precautions that are taken to prevent this situation from occurring. First, in fresh injuries only a half plaster is applied, i.e. a backslab that covers only half the limb but that will still immobilise the injury while leaving room for tissue swelling to occur (see p. 134). Second, the limb must be elevated to encourage tissue fluid to move, under gravity, away from the injured region. Coupled with these two steps should be observation of the limb for any changes in colour, warmth or sensation, in order to detect signs of neurovascular compromise as soon as possible.

Many patients will be discharged home rather than kept in hospital. Therefore, it is essential that they fully understand what they are looking for and the need to get in touch with the A & E unit if they do observe or experience anything unusual.

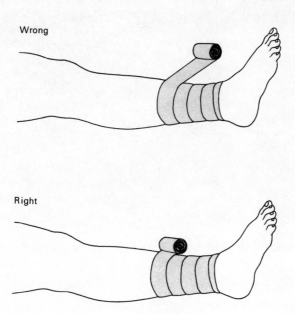

Fig. 7.1   The incorrect and the correct method of application of plaster bandage.

Because of the hazards of tissue swelling, it is essential in applying plaster not to make the POP too tight. The plaster bandage should be rolled onto the limb rather than a length of bandage unwound and then wrapped around the limb as shown in Fig. 7.1. This latter technique will make for a plaster that is too tight. This should also be remembered in applying the outer bandage to a backslab.

Limb Positioning

Once plastered, joints will remain in the same position for up to several weeks. It is essential, therefore, that they be plastered in the correct position. In the lower limb, the ankle should be at a perfect right angle. There should always be some 10° of flexion in the knee. In the upper limb, the usual position for the elbow is at 90° with the palm of the hand facing the body if the whole arm is to be immobilised. If the hand is to be placed in plaster (usually for a fractured metacarpal that has been manipulated), the position that should be adopted is the one shown in Fig. 7.2.

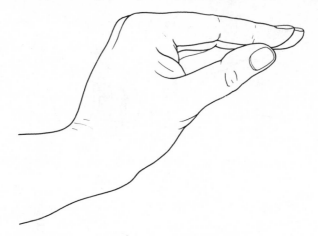

Fig. 7.2   Correct position for immobilisation of the hand.

Complete Setting Time

The plaster may seem very hard after some 5–10 minutes. However, it does take 48 hours to set fully and this must be explained to the patient. If it is a leg plaster, no weight must be allowed on the plaster for at least 48 hours or else a crumbling disintegration of the nurses' best efforts will be the result. Crutches must be provided together with instruction and demonstration on how to use them. Clothes should not be worn over a freshly applied POP as this will delay setting by interfering with the drying process.

<h2 style="text-align:center">Plaster of Paris Backslabs</h2>

In a fresh injury, a backslab is usually applied to allow room for swelling and to facilitate easy removal, if required, of the plaster. It consists of a slab of several layers of plaster bandage, cut to the required length and shape, and applied over a well-padded limb. It is bandaged in place while still wet by an open-weave cotton conforming bandage. The end of the bandage is secured with a further piece of plaster sticking it down to the plaster underneath, but not to the open padding as this would effectively be completing the plaster. (See Figs. 7.3, 7.4 and 7.5.)

Plaster Casts for Arm Injuries

Colles Cast

This type of cast will immobilise the wrist, but not the thumb. It is used for fractures of the distal radius. It should extend from just below the elbow to the metacarpophalangeal joints, leaving those joints free with a full range of movement. The thumb should be able to touch any of the fingers and the patient should have a reasonable grip. On the inner or palm-side of the wrist and hand (volar aspect), the plaster should extend no further than the proximal palmar crease. If the fracture has been manipulated, the position should be one of ulnar deviation and flexion. Plastering should commence with a 10 cm bandage turned twice around the proximal portion of the metacarpals and then passed twice between the thumb and index finger with a twisting motion before being continued up the arm in a spiral fashion. The plaster should be completed with a 15 cm bandage which should finish at the metacarpophalangeal joints.

Scaphoid Cast

Scaphoid fractures are exceptions to the rule about swelling, for there is usually very little associated with this injury. They can, therefore, go directly into a complete cast. Scaphoid fractures are notorious for not showing up on x-ray, but if the correct clinical finding of localised bony tenderness is noted over the scaphoid, the wrist should be plastered anyway. Very often the fracture will show on the second x-ray taken a week later, even though it did not show on the first.

The scaphoid cast is similar to the Colles cast, except that it immobilises the base of the thumb (the first metacarpophalangeal joint—mcp) and should leave the interphalangeal joint of the digit free. If there is a fracture through the base of the thumb involving the mcp joint, it is called a Bennett's fracture and requires the interphalangeal joint to be included in the plaster.

Padding is, therefore, required around the thumb as well as the rest of the wrist and forearm. The plaster should be started with a 7.5 cm bandage turned twice around the proximal portion of the metacarpals before being taken twice around the base of the thumb, and completed with a 15 cm bandage. The patient should be able to touch finger tips with thumb when the scaphoid cast is complete.

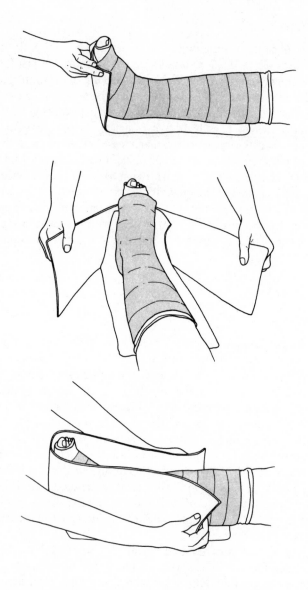

Fig. 7.3   Backslab for ankle/foot injuries.

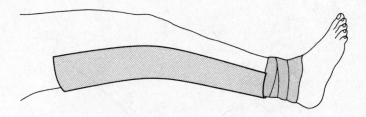

2x20cm backslabs overlapping at the back of the leg
Finish above the ankle which must be well padded
Knee flexed at 10°

Fig. 7.4 Backslab for knee injuries.

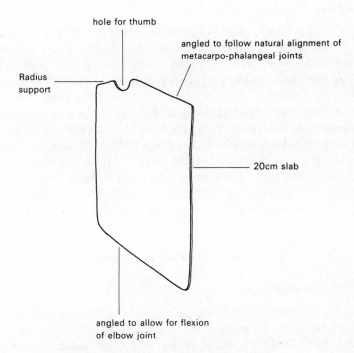

hole for thumb

angled to follow natural alignment of
metacarpo-phalangeal joints

Radius
support

20cm slab

angled to allow for flexion
of elbow joint

Fig. 7.5 Backslab for wrist injuries.

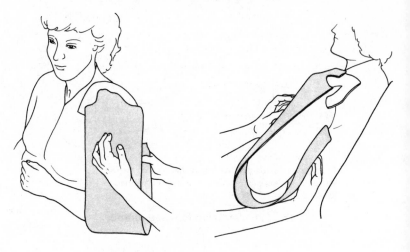

Fig. 7.6   Hanging U slab for humerus fracture.

Full Arm Plasters

If the elbow is to be immobilised, the plaster will need to extend to the top of the upper arm. Particular attention should be paid to the area of the brachial artery to ensure there is no constriction in this region. Care should also be taken that the plaster is not causing discomfort under the axilla. It is usual to plaster the elbow at 90° with the palm of the hand facing the body. The wrist may be left out of the cast or included, depending on the injury. For example, if a Smith's fracture of the wrist is to be treated conservatively, it is typically done so in a plaster that will immobilise the elbow as well as the wrist due to the risk of the fracture slipping if the forearm is allowed to rotate, a movement that occurs at the elbow. Conversely, a supracondylar fracture of the humerus can be treated by leaving the wrist joint free, outside the plaster. (See Fig. 7.6.)

Plaster Casts for Leg Injuries

Below Knee Plasters

For a simple below knee plaster, a 20 cm bandage should be used, starting at the base of the toes and working up the leg to finish just below the head of the fibula. The ankle should be at a right angle. Two or three bandages will be required depending on the size of the leg. If a walking heel is to be added, scraps of plaster should be used to fill in the hollow that will be present on the sole of the plaster due to the arch of the foot. There must be a true, flat surface to attach the walking heel in the correct position. It should be secured using a 10 cm bandage woven in a figure of 8 fashion. The actual walking surfaces, however, should be left free of plaster. The walking heel needs to be centrally aligned if the patient is to be able to walk comfortably and safely.

Long Leg Cylinders

A long leg cylinder is usually applied for fractures of the tibia and fibula or injuries involving the knee. It should extend from just above the malleoli to the top of the thigh, and will benefit from having backslabs incorporated in it to give added strength. For fractures of the tibia and fibula, it is often easier if the plaster is applied in two stages. First, a below knee plaster should be applied to immobilise the fracture; then the cast should be completed by incorporating the knee and thigh in a second stage. For knee injuries, the idea of a two stage plaster is also relevant, with the knee first being immobilised with a full leg backslab which, when set, can be plastered over to convert into a reinforced cylinder. The ankle should have plenty of padding to protect the malleoli and achilles tendon area; the knee must be in a slight flexion of about 5 to 10°.

Discharging the Patient with a Plaster of Paris Cast

When an individual is discharged with a POP, they are confronted with a series of real problems in self-care. Reference to Orem's model of nursing (see p. 32) shows that the patient has a series of universal self-care demands to fulfil. Now, with the handicap of a POP, there are specific problems which require self-care. These are the health deviancy areas of structure (the cast itself), function (the immobilised limb) and behaviour (how does the patient react mentally to immobility?). A substantial amount of knowledge and understanding is required if the patient is to successfully achieve self-care in all these areas. It is the A & E nurses' responsibility to teach the patient what is required in order that self-care may be carried out effectively.

The first health deviancy area to consider is structure. Plaster of Paris will crumble if it becomes wet. The patient should, therefore, be instructed to keep the plaster dry, and should be told why this is necessary. The problems of swelling within the cast and the neurovascular complications that can occur due to compression of blood vessels and nerves should be carefully explained to the patient. The patient should also be instructed about the possible signs of problems—swollen digits, discolouration and altered sensation—and about elevating the limb. A sling can be used for the arm; for the leg, the patient should sit with the foot higher than the level of the heart.

The final major problem concerning the plaster itself stems from the fact that it takes 48 hours to set properly. This is not much of a problem for arm plasters, but if it is a leg cast that the patient will eventually be allowed to walk on, it is important that the patient understand that no weight can be taken by the plaster for 48 hours. Crutches must be supplied together with instruction on how to use them. The patient should be asked to demonstrate their competence in using the crutches before being allowed to leave the department.

The second health deviancy involves function; stiffness will develop as a result of immobilisation. The patient should, therefore, be encouraged to retain maximum movement in the limb by having various exercises demonstrated. For example, if a wrist plaster has been applied, finger exercises should be taught to the patient to maintain both extension and flexion; the importance of keeping the elbow and shoulder joints mobile should also be made clear. This is of special importance in elderly patients whose joints stiffen up very quickly.

The final area of health deviancy is that of behaviour. Lack of mobility may make some patients depressed or frustrated. This potential problem should be explored with the patient in advance in order that he or she be mentally prepared to cope with it.

Nurses need to consider that the plaster affects the whole person and not just the single limb. An example of this is the 75 year old lady who has to use a zimmer frame to get about. If this patient sustains a fracture of the arm, which is then placed in plaster, it may make it impossible for her to use the zimmer frame. There will no longer be a balance between rest and activity. Social interaction will be severely limited, and if the patient tries to mobilise without a zimmer, she will be exposed to a much more hazardous environment. There is, therefore, a major deficit in self-care which nurses must try to fill by either involving family or community services; if that fails, an admission to hospital may be required.

Before discharging a patient home in plaster, the A & E nurse must consider whether self-care can be achieved in terms of the universal requirements associated with everyday living, and in terms of specific problems relating directly to the plaster. Orem's model of nursing makes an elegant framework around which to plan for the patient's care after discharge. Initially the A & E nurse fills a partly compensatory role by immobilising the injury for the patient (thereby meeting the patient's self-care deficit). Then the nurse moves on to the educative/advisory role in preparing the patient for self-care on discharge.

Chapter 8

SOFT TISSUE INJURY

Pathology

Soft tissue injury can either be closed, as in bruising or a ligament sprain, or open, in which case some sort of wound will be present. The wounds seen in A & E are rather different from the surgical incisions that the nurse will have encountered elsewhere: A & E wounds can be in all shapes and sizes, and are all caused by non-sterile agents, with an accompanying high risk of infection. The following summary of wounds commonly seen in A & E will be of use as an introduction:

1. *Laceration.* A linear cut in the skin, usually superficial but may involve deep structures.

2. *Crush injury.* Fingers and toes are the most commonly involved. There may be a fracture of the bone underneath which will, therefore, be an open fracture. The force of the impact causes the soft tissue to burst open; a very painful injury with much swelling involved.

3. *Penetrating wound.* A narrow but deeply penetrating track is involved. The cause can be anything from treading on a nail to a stabbing or gunshot wound.

4. *Abrasions.* A superficial but very painful injury. Dirt and grit is commonly ingrained or tatooed into the skin and has to be removed by scrubbing.

5. *Bites.* Ragged wounds are produced by bites and have a very high risk of infection. The most infective bite of all is a human bite, which for this reason should never be sutured.

6. *Degloving injury.* If a force is involved that is parallel to the skin, layers of tissue maybe torn away, exposing a whole area of deeper structures.

7. *Burns.* See next chapter.

The normal healing process of wounds involves the formation initially of granulation tissue and then of scar tissue which, by virtue of its contractile properties, closes the wound. An impaired blood supply, infection or the presence of foreign material will all delay or prevent healing. The aim in A & E, therefore, is to thoroughly clean the wound, removing foreign material and reducing the risk of infection, and then to close the wound so as to promote rapid healing with the minimum of scar formation and infection risk.

The most feared pathogens are the anaerobic Clostridium family. *Clostridium tetani* gives rise to tetanus, and *Clostridium welchii* and *Clostridium sporagenes* are involved in gas gangrene. The spores of these organisms are found in the soil, and the fact that they are anaerobic means that they can live without free atmospheric oxygen. Therefore, if they are present in a wound that is closed over, they will thrive.

Tetanus is characterised by the toxins which are released by the *Clostridium tetani* attacking the nervous system. The result is severe muscle spasm which could be fatal once the muscles of respiration become involved. In established cases, therefore, the treatment involves long-term ventilatory support.

In gas gangrene, putrefactive changes occur within damaged or dead tissue. The clostridia are responsible for forming various hydrogen gasses which escape into the tissue planes, giving the characteristic odour. The gas increases the pressure in the tissues surrounding the wound. This further impairs blood supply. Meanwhile, the toxins released by the bacteria cause a severe toxaemia. The condition is extremely painful and carries a high mortality rate.

A wide variety of other pathogens cause wound sepsis. As the patient in most cases is going home after treatment, it is important that the signs of infection be carefully explained. The patient should be given instructions to return should there be any signs of infection, such as pain, swelling, redness or inflammation tracking up the limb along the line of a vein.

The elderly have very fragile skin, and suturing is not necessarily the best means of closing wounds in this case as sutures may simply cut through the skin. The pre-tibial flap laceration is a common injury seen in elderly ladies and is best treated by the use of steristrips rather than sutures. If it is proximally based (see Fig. 8.1), there is a good chance of healing. The distally based flap, however, has a very poor blood supply and often necroses, and a skin grafting operation is needed.

In dealing with gunshot or shrapnel injuries, it is important to determine the velocity of the projectile. If the velocity exceeds that of sound, the particle is supersonic and is defined as a high velocity missile. It will behave in a very different way from a subsonic particle (a particle travell-

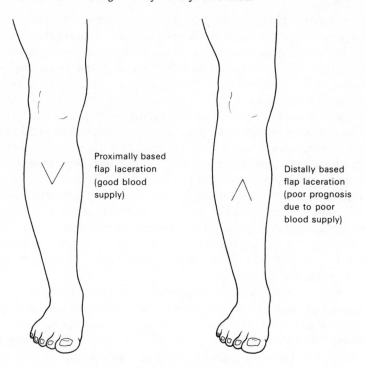

Fig. 8.1   Pretibial flap laceration.

ing below the speed of sound). For example, the muzzle velocity of the average handgun is some 550 feet per second. The velocity of sound is 1100 feet per second. A modern military rifle, on the other hand, has a muzzle velocity of about 2500 feet per second and the Colt Armolite exceeds 3000 feet per second. At these supersonic speeds, there is a high pressure shock wave preceding the projectile and, in its wake, there is a vacuum. The result on hitting the human body is an instantaneous pressure wave, causing catastrophic damage. This is followed by the vacuum which sucks gross contamination deep into the wound. A volume of tissue roughly equal to that of a football may be destroyed by a single bullet, with only a tiny entrance and exit wound to show for it. Bone is shattered, muscle and soft tissue infarcted and blood vessels destroyed, simply due to the pressure wave and without any physical contact with the projectile.

Of the closed soft tissue injuries, one of the most common categories are the sprains. These consist of ligament injury where the ligament is grossly intact, but some individual fibres have been torn. The result is painful and associated with a lot of swelling, but the joint is stable. Bruising can have serious consequences because in areas such as the foot and calf there may be little room for expansion to accommodate the extra tissue fluid. Pressure levels can rise to such a point that the microcirculation is impaired and serious neurovascular complications can develop.

Other commonly seen injuries include trauma to cartilage and bursae. In the knee, a tear of one of the semilunar cartilages is commonly associated with a twisting movement when the knee is flexed, resulting in the patient's knee locking in a flexed position. Repeated wear and tear on the bursae of the elbow or knee can lead to inflammation, swelling and pain, the so-called housemaid's knee or tennis elbow.

Although not traumatic in origin, the A & E department is commonly visited by patients with a wide variety of skin lesions. Table 8.1 makes a useful summary of the more common rashes and their origins.

Assessment

In assessing wounds, the nurse will often be confronted by a very distressed relative and/or patient clutching a bloodstained rag to the wound. The effect of the sight of blood can be very dramatic for some people. Therefore, the nurse needs a calm, reassuring manner in order to obtain a history. The nurse needs to find out what caused the injury, how, when and how much blood loss there has been. It is worth remembering, however, that the lay person is prone to over-exaggerate blood loss.

Taking a pad of gauze, the next thing the nurse should do is to examine the wound itself, carefully removing the patient's own first aid dressing. The nurse should look for the depth and extent of the wound, see if any deep structures such as tendons are visible and if so whether they are damaged, note any contamination and, if bleeding occurs, note whether it is pulsatile and therefore arterial in nature. Finally the degree of pain felt by the patient should be assessed.

The assessment should then move on to the area distal to the wound to see if there is any evidence of damage to structures such as tendons and nerves. The nurse should test sensation and movement with this consideration in mind and also note the colour and warmth of the skin.

The psychological state of the patient should be assessed as the sight of blood can be a very frightening experience; the possibility of either the patient or relative fainting as a result should always be kept in mind.

When there has been significant blood loss, or a penetrating injury, it

Table 8.1   Common rashes seen in A & E

Disease	Chief Complaint	History
Herpes Simplex Type 1 (Cold Sore)	Usually around mouth or nose; group of vessicles rupture leaving painful ulcer with yellow crust.	Colds, fever, menstruation or overexposure to sunlight may precede outbreak.
Herpes Simplex Type 2 (Genital Herpes)	Small grouped vessicles around genitals and mouth.	Sexual contact with infected person.
Herpes Zoster (Shingles)	Grouped vessicles or crusted lesions along nerve root.	Chicken pox, reactivation of virus may cause attack.
Verucae (Warts)	Slightly raised papules.	Previous history of warts.
Rubeola (Measles)	Rash begins with macules on hairline, neck and cheeks, spreads downwards over rest of body. Appears 2–4 days after other symptoms, lasts 4–5 days.	Exposure to infected person 10–14 days previously. Cold, cough fever before rash.
Rubella (German Measles)	Maculopapular rash begins on face, spreads to trunk.	Exposure to infected person 14–21 days previously. Adolescents have malaise, fever, anorexia and headaches before rash.
Varicella (Chicken Pox)	Appears first on trunk, spreads to face and scalp. Small red papules and clear vessicles on red base which break and dry leaving a crust. Itching.	Exposure to infected person 13–21 days ago. Malaise and anorexia before rash.
Tinea corporis (Ringworm)	Intense itching. Round red scaly lesions, central area heals while lesion continues outward.	Exposure to infected animals or persons. Most common in children.
Tinea capitis (Scalp Ringworm)	Mild itching, small spreading papules cause hair loss.	Exposure to infected persons.

Table derived from Holderman, M.C. (1984): *Nursing 84*, November. pp 22–23. Philadelphia, Pa.: Springhouse Corp.

is essential to record vital signs and then monitor them as necessary as hypovolaemia can develop very quickly. Remember that a small entry wound in the case of a penetrating wound can conceal devastating injury within.

The patient's anti-tetanus status should also be ascertained, together with any other information relevant to wound healing, such as whether the patient is a diabetic or on steroid therapy.

In assessing closed soft tissue injuries, first a history should be obtained. Then the nurse should move on to look at the injury. It needs examining for localised bony tenderness, which would raise the possibility of a fracture, and for swelling, pain and degree of function. It is important to know how rapidly the existing amount of swelling occurred so that a reasonable estimate can be made of future swelling and, therefore, whether there is a significant risk of neurovascular compromise.

A common type of lesion that is presented at A & E is the wound that has become infected because the person did not seek treatment at the time. In addition, people present with a wide range of abscesses, some of which can be extremely painful. In assessing the patient, the nurse should obtain a history of how long the problem has existed and of any likely precipitating factor. The area should be examined for signs of the infection spreading such as a red prominent track along the line of a vein or the swelling of lymph nodes. Due to the association of infective lesions with diabetes, the patient should have a routine urinalysis performed for glucose. Temperature and pulse should also be recorded to assess the degree of systemic involvement.

Intervention

Control Bleeding

The first intervention is to stop any bleeding. This may be done by direct pressure over the wound with a firm dressing—initially this can be held by hand, but a firm bandage will suffice once the bleeding has been stopped—and by elevating the injury, for example, by using a roller towel and a drip stand for a hand or arm injury. Injuries as extreme as traumatic amputations of limbs may be dealt with in this way. There is no indication for the use of a tourniquet in A & E other than to provide a temporary bloodless field for a brief examination of the wound.

Cleaning the Wound

Whether it is a major wound that will require repair in theatre or a minor wound that can be dealt with in A & E, it will need cleaning out thoroughly. If the wound is major, irrigation with a litre of normal saline in A & E is recommended. This can be followed by a dressing of saline soaks and iodine to keep the tissue in the best condition possible for theatre, where a formal toilet and debridement will take place. The aim is, in addition to a thorough toilet of the wound to wash out all contamination, to surgically remove any dead or dubious tissue which may act as a focus for infection (e.g. gas gangrene). The surgeon may leave badly contaminated wounds open for 3 days after surgery, covering them with only a light gauze dressing. Only when absolutely sure that there is no evidence of sepsis, will the surgeon proceed to a delayed primary suture. This procedure is mandatory for all high velocity missile wounds.

An excellent agent for cleaning wounds in A & E is hydrogen peroxide. The chemical reaction which occurs when a wound is irrigated with hydrogen peroxide loosens contamination and flushes it free of the wound. The wound should then be given a generous cleansing with an antiseptic solution such as Savlodil.

Abrasions demand special attention as grit may be tattooed into the wound. If left there, it will cause infection and possibly a permanent disfiguring mark. The vigorous use of a scrubbing brush and hydrogen peroxide is the only effective way to remove such grit. Needless to say this is a very painful procedure and the patient should have the benefit of either a general anaesthetic, Entonox and local anaesthesia, or IV pethidine.

Wound Closure

The two main techniques used in A & E for wound closure are suturing and steristripping. Both techniques have certain points in common; the closing agent should always be applied at right angles to the wound, skin edges should never be inverted (turned under) as this delays healing, and the tension in the skin around the wound should be evenly distributed.

According to Orem's model of nursing, suturing may be thought of as a normal part of the nurse's role as it fulfils the patient's health deviancy self-care demands in terms of structure, i.e. closing a wound. The nurse will find the technique illustrated in Fig. 8.2 to be effective in dealing with most wounds that will require suturing in A & E.

If more than one stitch is required, the area should first be infiltrated with local anaesthetic which should be introduced via a needle inserted parallel to the wound and injected as the needle and syringe are gradually withdrawn. Lignocaine 2% is the agent of choice. However, in a very vascular area, such as the scalp, where bleeding often proves a problem, lignocaine with adrenaline may be used. Such a solution should never be used on a finger or toe as the vasoconstrictor effects of adrenaline are so great that peripheral gangrene may result.

The needle should be firmly gripped half-way to one-third along its length by the needle holders. When the needle is introduced into the skin, it is important that the wrist be rotated in alignment with the curvature of the needle, otherwise the needle will be bent. The needle should enter some 4 mm from the wound edge and exit the same distance from the opposite side of the wound. Dissecting forceps may be used to hold the wound edge to facilitate passing the needle through.

The knot is tied as shown in the diagram, some three turns being needed, each in opposite direction from its predecessor. Each stitch needs to be about 3 mm from its neighbour. In cutting the stitch, the nurse should remember that a colleague will have to remove that stitch in a few days time—3 days for faces, 5 days for scalps, 7 days for elsewhere. For faces, 5–0 size suture material is usually used; 4–0 is used elsewhere although if considerable force is involved (e.g. over a knee), 3–0 may be used. Scalps are also often sutured with 3–0.

Steristrips are simply thin strips of adhesive paper (see Fig. 8.3). They are suitable for many wounds, do not require local anaesthetic and leave less scar than sutures. They cannot, however, be applied to hairy areas such as the scalp, and if the wound is over a joint, they will probably be pulled apart by tension in the skin as movement occurs.

The skin on either side of a wound should be prepared by having tinct. benzene spray wiped over it to improve its adhesive properties. For most wounds 3 mm strips will suffice; 6 mm or 12 mm are available for bigger wounds. The strips should be attached while the tinct. benzene is still tacky, first to one side of the wound. The wound is then pulled together and the strip stuck down onto the skin the other side. In large or ragged wounds, it may be necessary to perform a two stage closure, using some strips initially to approximate the wound edges, and then proceeding to fully close the wound with further strips, removing the first strips in the process.

A gap should be left between strips to allow for drainage of any fluid from the wound. Finally, anchoring strips should be applied parallel to the wound to evenly distribute skin tension.

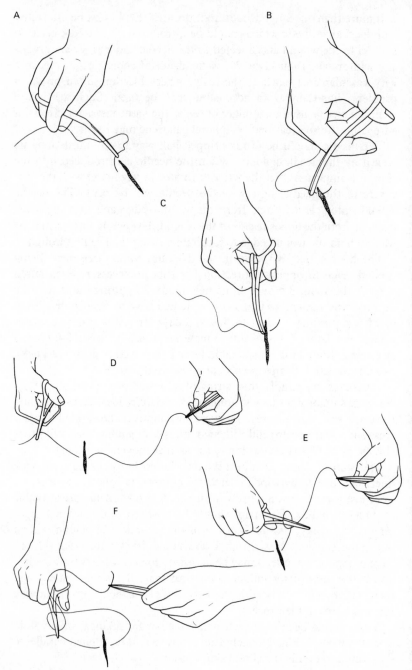

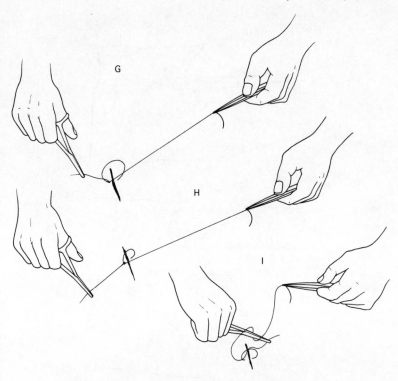

Fig. 8.2 Suturing technique.
(a) Note that needle holders grasp the needle approximately one-third along the needle and not at the end. The point of the needle is perpendicular to the skin at point of entry. The point of entry should be 3–4 mm from wound.
(b) By rotating the wrist, bring the needle through and out of the wound.
(c) Re-enter on the opposite edge of the wound, rotating the wrist to bring the needle out 3–4 mm from the opposite side of the wound.
(d) Pull the suture through the wound, ready for tying the knot.
(e) Start tying the knot by making a loop with the needle holders.
(f) Grasp the end of the suture.
(g) Pull the end of the suture through the loop.
(h) Pull it firmly but not too tightly, laying the knot to one side of the wound.
(i) Then repeat this twice, looping in the opposite direction on each occasion.

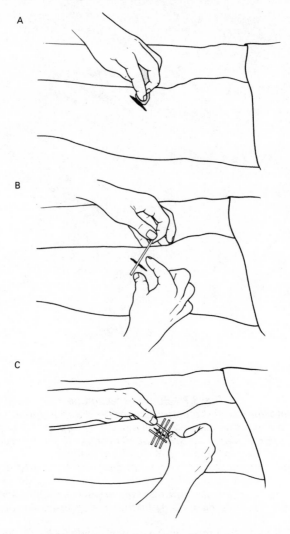

Fig. 8.3 Steristripping technique.
(a) After a thorough cleaning of the wound, wipe the skin on either side of the wound with tinct benzene.
(b) Pinch the skin edges together and lay the strips across it.
(c) Leave gaps between the strips and finish by laying two anchor strips parallel to the wound.

Minor scalp lacerations can be effectively dealt with by simply tying together strands of hair from either side of the wound.

Dressing the Wound

The aim is to have an occlusive, sterile dressing which will have the minimum interference with limb function, will remain in place for the required period, and can be removed with the minimum discomfort to the patient.

Plain dry gauze should not be in direct contact with the wound itself because it absorbs blood and exudate to form a hard, adherent mass that can be very difficult and painful to remove. One of the non-adherent proprietary dressings should be used in contact with the wound itself, backed if necessary by layers of gauze. If an area of tissue loss (e.g. an abrasion) is to be dressed, a paraffin impregnated gauze should also be used. Preferably it should be one that has an antiseptic such as chlorhexidine incorporated in it (e.g. Bactigras). There is no extra advantage to be gained from using the more expensive antibiotic impregnated gauzes.

The dressing may be secured to the skin with a hypoallergenic tape (e.g. Micropore) applied longitudinally as any swelling may give rise to circulatory impairment if there is a circumferential constriction around the limb or digit.

The use of an elasticated tube type of dressing (e.g. Tubigrip) is recommended, rather than the traditional crêpe bandage, to complete the dressing. It is cheaper, easier to apply, gives a more even pressure over the limb with no risk of the wrinkles that can cause skin problems, and will stay in place far more effectively than a crêpe bandage. Bandages applied to legs and ankles invariably fall down in 24 hours.

Finger dressings can be retained with a tubular bandage (e.g. Tubinette), the important point being to tie the bandage at the wrist, and not at the base of the digit, in order to avoid the risk of circulatory impairment (see Fig. 8.4). If swelling is anticipated, the hand should be placed in a high arm sling (see Fig. 8.5).

Head wounds may need a pressure bandage even after suture, a size F Tubigrip, 10 cm long, worn as a headband provides a very simple and effective solution to the problem, rather than the intricacies of head bandaging so beloved of the first aid manuals. Similarly the elasticated tube bandages (e.g. Netelast) provide a better means of securing dressings to the trunk than does the traditional body bandage.

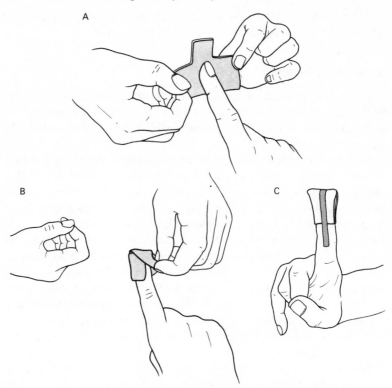

Fig. 8.4   Application of a fingertip dressing.
(a) Note the 'T' shape cut out of dressing pad.
(b) Secure the dressing longitudinally with the tape.
Circumferential taping is a potential tournique for a freshly injured finger.
(c) The dressing is ready for the application of a tubular bandage.

Tetanus Vaccination

The effectiveness of the anti-tetanus immunisation programme in the UK can be judged from the fact that there are no more than one or two dozen cases per year compared to the death toll from tetanus of a million or more per year in the Third World.

The adsorbed tetanus toxoid that is given to patients in A & E units is a form of active immunisation in that it stimulates the patient to manufacture their own antibodies. A second injection is required 6 weeks after the first to continue the process and raise immunity to safe levels. A third injection is given to complete the course at twelve months; this will

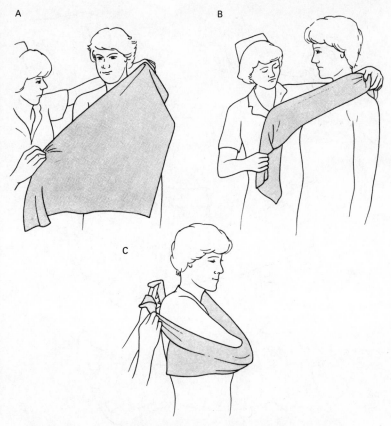

Fig. 8.5 Application of a high arm sling.
(a) This shows the position of the sling. Ensure that the hand that
is injured is placed on the opposite shoulder.
(b) Wrap the sling around the arm and hand. Pin to ensure that
the hand is enclosed.
(c) Tie the sling at the back.

maintain antibody levels for 5 years (some authorities say 10) before a
further booster is needed. Anti-tetanus injections are a normal part of
the childhood injections received in the UK. Therefore, any child that
has had its triple injections as an infant will have received anti-tetanus
cover.

If the patient states that they have never received any anti-tetanus immunisation, it is possible to give passive immunity in the form of the
appropriate human immunoglobulin if the medical staff assess the risk
as being significant.

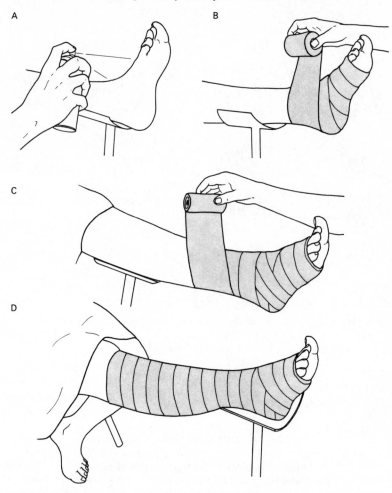

Fig. 8.6 Application of elastoplast strapping for a sprained ankle.
(a) Spray skin with tinct benzene. Spray from base of toes to head of fibula.
(b) Commencing from base of toes, wrap elastoplast in a spiral fashion round the foot, then in 'figure of eight' style around the ankle.
(c) Wrap the strapping spiral fashion up the rest of the leg, overlapping as far as the yellow line on the strapping.
(d) The strapping should be complete from the base of the toes to level with the head of the fibula. The foot should be in a right angle position.

Closed Soft Tissue Injury

The usual aim is to treat closed soft tissue injury conservatively by rest and support. Swelling can be reduced by elevation and ice packs if necessary. Gradually the area can be mobilised as pain and swelling ease off. Either elastoplast strapping (Fig. 8.6) or tubigrip may be used to lend support to the injury in this stage. If a sprain of the ankle is so severe as to prevent full weight-bearing, consideration should be given to plaster of Paris to immobilise the injury. Crêpe bandage is of little effective use.

Abscesses

Abscesses are commonly treated surgically by the casualty officer, under general or local anaesthesia. The appropriate preparation of the patient is, therefore, required in line with hospital procedure, together with a full explanation of what is to happen and how long the procedure will take.

It is essential after incision and drainage that the cavity be carefully dressed with a non-adherent dressing and sufficient gauze to absorb any further exudate. The actual cavity is usually packed with ribbon gauze soaked in a chlorine-based antiseptic such as Eusol. If the infected area involves the hand, a high arm sling is needed to minimise swelling.

The patient will usually be discharged with a course of antibiotics and analgesics. The nurse should ensure that the patient understands the label on the bottles and knows which are the analgesics and which the antibiotics. The patient also must understand the need to complete the full course of antibiotics even if the infection appears to clear up before completion. The nurse can remember that the patient's care from now on will be self-care until they return for their next appointment when the nurse will be able to check progress on the healing of the abscess. If necessary, patients may be given dressings to take home and may change the dressing themselves, providing correct instruction is given in A & E first. The value of developing a self-care approach to nursing in the mode of Orem is evident from just this one common example of A & E care.

Self-care

It is important that the patient be instructed in self-care of the injury before discharge. Key points include the need for elevation, keeping the

Date Time	Potential Problem	Patient Goal	Dead-line	Nursing Intervention	Evaluation: Were assessment and intervention carried out as in Nursing Intervention?			
					Yes	No	N/A	Effectiveness in meeting self-care deficit.
				1. Complete Standard Nursing Assessment				
				2. Obtain data specific to chief complaint: history, time since injury, size, depth and degree of contamination of wound, function/sensation distally, swelling.				
				3. Complete Standard Nursing Intervention.				
	Patient unable to prevent wound bleeding.	Bleeding from wound will stop.		4.1 Direct pressure to wound. 4.2 Elevate limb.				
	Body defences unable to prevent infection.	Wound will not become infected.		5.1 Irrigate with saline/H_2O_2. 5.2 Saline/Iodine dressings. 5.3 Prepare for theatre. 5.4 Cleanse with H_2O_2/antiseptic. 5.5 Close wound. 5.6 Dressing. 5.7 Give anti-tetanus immunisation. 5.8 Education in wound self-care.				
	Pain which the patient cannot relieve.	Patient will feel relief of pain.		6.1 Give Entonox. 6.2 Reduce swelling (elevation). 6.3 Support dressing (elastoplast etc.). 6.4 Immobilise joint (POP).				
	Patient's wound remains open.	Wound will be closed.		7.1 Suture. 7.2 Steristrip. 7.3 Tie hair.				
	Patient develops hypovolaemia.	Patient's BP remains normal.		See 3 and 4.				
	Patient will faint.	Patient will not faint.		8.1 Minimise sight of blood. 8.2 Offer psychological support. 8.3 Lie patient down.				

Fig. 8.7 Standard Care Plan: Soft Tissue Injury

dressing dry and clean, the length of time until dressing or suture removal, and instructions about how to remove the dressings or where to go to get the sutures removed. The patient should be alerted about the signs of infection and instructed to return immediately if there is any suspicion of infection. If a full course of tetanus is required, the patient should be given a card with the dates of the next two injections and the nurse should emphasise the importance of the follow-up injections. In this case, the nurse is filling the educative/supportive role of Orem after the partly compensatory role which will have been filled at an earlier stage during treatment.

Evaluation

All dressings performed by junior staff should be checked before the patient is discharged, for if they are done incorrectly, they go home wrong and remain wrong.

In many respects, the only real evaluation of treatment is if the patient returns or not. If the patient does not return, the assumption is that the nursing interventions have been successful. If the patient does return with a problem, however, the nursing staff should try to see how nursing care could have been better carried out. This will benefit other patients in the future.

In order to evaluate the effectiveness of self-care instruction, it is essential to question the patient to see that they fully understand what has been taught.

Chapter 9

THE BURNT PATIENT IN A & E

Pathology

The key factors in burn pathology are the area of the burn, the depth of the burn, and any special areas of the body, such as the respiratory tract, that are involved.

Area

The burnt area will almost immediately begin to lose fluid which is very similar to plasma in its composition. If sufficient fluid is lost from the burn, hypovolaemic shock will develop. The area of the burn is, therefore, crucial as it determines the volume of fluid lost. Area may be estimated using Wallace's Rule of 9 (see Fig. 9.1).

As a rule of thumb it may be assumed that in burns of 15% of surface area or greater in adults, and 10% or greater in children, hypovolaemia will develop. In these cases, therefore, the patient will need an IVI. If such an infusion is not commenced and the hypovolaemia not vigorously treated, the outcome may be fatal.

In reading about burns, the nurse may be confused by the different statements that are made about the type of fluid that should be used to correct hypovolaemia from burns. This is because there is a marked difference of opinion among the various specialists in the field. The basic requirements in the burn patient are salt and water in such a form as will stay in the circulation. Sodium chloride is lost in great quantities in the burn exudate; on the other hand, ordinary solutions such as normal saline or Dextrose 5% will rapidly leak into the extracellular fluid, only 20% remaining in the plasma within a matter of minutes. The sort of IV fluid required is, therefore, either Dextran 70 (dextran in saline) or plasma protein faction (PPF), both of which are made up of large molecules and thus will remain in the circulation, and both of which contain sodium chloride.

Fluid loss from a burn continues for over 24 hours after injury. This is of significance in planning dressings for patients that are to be dis-

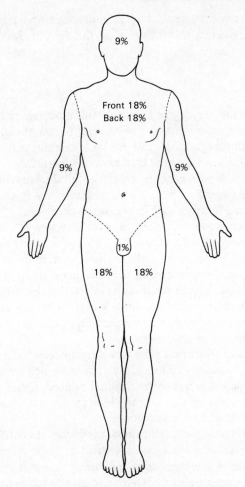

Fig. 9.1   Wallace's Rule of 9 for estimating area of burns.

charged home with relatively minor burns. For the major burn requiring in-patient treatment, the continual fluid loss has to be taken into account in working out an IVI regime. Various formulae are used in this connection, one of the best known being the Mount Vernon formula which calculates a unit volume of fluid from the patient's size and the area burnt.

Unit volume = Area burnt (%) × Patient's weight (kg) ÷ 2

This unit volume of fluid is then administered in blocks of 4 hours, two blocks of 6 hours and one block of 12 hours, measured from the time of the burn and subject to adjustment in the light of the patient's condition.

Depth

The 1st, 2nd and 3rd degree burns classifications are to be avoided as they are imprecise terms that can mean different things to different people. It is more appropriate and precise to describe the depth of burns as either full thickness, partial thickness or superficial.

A full thickness burn is one in which the full thickness of the skin has been destroyed (see Fig. 9.2). The appearance is a typically dull grey area, or in flame burns, a dark brown or black. Because the nerve endings have been destroyed, there is usually a loss of sensation. The remaining tissue is hard and leathery. This poses a special problem in circumferential burns because the inelastic surface tissue will act as a tourniquet around the limb, within which there will be swelling due to the burn oedema. The result is occlusion of the circulation, gangrene and loss of the limb, unless the limb is excised longitudinally through the eschar tissue to allow room for expansion and for the release of pressure. This is known as escharrotomy.

Healing of a full thickness burn occurs by the formation of scar tissue, which is both unsightly and inelastic. The inelasticity will give rise to loss of function and severe contractures. The need, therefore, is to treat full thickness burns by skin grafting in order to retain maximum function and avoid contracture formation.

If the burn is only partial thickness, then areas of epithelium survive around hair follicles and sweat glands. This permits the re-epithelialisation of the burnt area, providing that it is kept free from infection. Skin grafting is, therefore, not usually required and healing should occur with a full range of movement. Partial thickness burns usually leave the nerve endings intact, therefore, they may be differentiated from full thickness burns by a pin prick sensation test. Scalds and flash burns are typically partial thickness.

Superficial burns involve a reddening only of the most superficial layers. This is known as erythema and is of minor importance compared to the other two types so far discussed. In estimating burn areas, erythema should be excluded.

One final type of burn that should be mentioned is the burn due to electricity. It is characterised by a small surface wound where the current entered the body, but within there may be major damage with

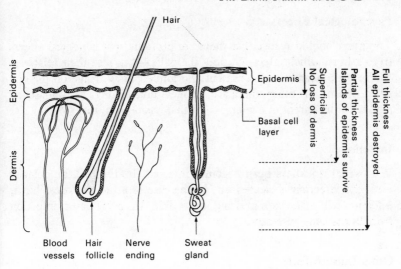

Fig. 9.2   Depth of burns.

burns extending down to the bone and involving structures such as tendons, muscles and nerves. The potential effect of the electric current on the heart should be the first focus of nursing and medical attention.

Special Areas Affected by Burns

Oedema of the face and neck can have serious implications for the airway. Inhalation of flames or hot gasses will cause burn oedema in the respiratory tract itself. The threat of an occluded airway is very real in such cases and an early tracheotomy or intubation, if possible, is indicated.

Facial oedema will quickly make it impossible for the patient to open their eyes. This has two implications; first, if the eyes are to be examined properly, they must be examined immediately, and second, the patient may fear that their sight has been lost altogether, when the problem is simply that they cannot open their eyes.

Immobilisation of hands in bulky dressings will lead to long-term problems of joint stiffness. For this reason, the 'Flamazine bag' dressing is recommended for burnt hands rather than more traditional methods (see Fig. 9.3 on p. 166). Flamazine is silver sulphadiazine, a very effective antibacterial agent.

Psychological Effects

The nurse should realise that there are profound psychological effects from a burn which affect not only the patient but also their relatives. There is the fear of disfigurement and altered body image on the one hand, and on the other, there are the inevitable feelings of guilt associated with the parent of a young child that has been burnt.

Infection

If a partial thickness burn becomes infected, healing will be delayed until the infection is cleared up. In the case of a full thickness burn, infection will make skin grafting impossible. In severe cases, infection from burns can cause death.

Other Later Effects

After the patient has moved to the ward, complications can develop. These include renal failure, toxaemia, anaemia, paralytic ileus, and in the case of children 'burn encephalopathy'. These complications can combine to make the burns victim an extremely challenging person to care for.

Assessment

Assessment of the burns victim starts with the airway. The nurse should note whether the burns involve the face and neck areas, and whether there is any evidence of the patient having inhaled flames or hot gas. Such evidence would include soot in the nasal passages or blistering around the mouth and lips.

It is important to obtain a history of the accident—what caused the burn, the time the burn occurred and what, if any, first aid has been applied. The next point to determine is how much pain the patient is feeling. Some burns cause remarkably little pain; ironically they are usually the more severe full thickness burns, but other burns can be extremely painful.

The area of the burn should be estimated, using Wallace's Rule of 9 (see Fig. 9.1). This rule divides the body area up into multiples of 9%. For small areas, the area of the patient's hand can be taken as 1% of the body area.

The last point to estimate is the depth of the burn. The appearance will give some clue: a full thickness burn is typically a dull grey colour with tough leathery eschar tissue; a partial thickness burn is usually red or pink in colour. Sensation is absent in the full thickness burn but present in a partial thickness burn. This may be tested for with the pin prick method.

A sketch of the burn is a useful means of recording its extent; areas of suspected full thickness burn can be shaded in and labelled as such.

Baseline observations are important to monitor the circulatory status of the patient and to detect any signs of hypovolaemic shock at the earliest stage. They should be repeated as frequently as the patient's condition indicates.

The psychological effects of the burn on the patient and on the family should be assessed, especially where young children are involved. Is the mother hostile and defensive, or anxious and expressing feelings of guilt? One important aspect that has to be assessed is whether the child's injuries match the story of the parent as burns constitute one of the commonest forms of child abuse.

In electrical burns, it is important to take an ECG and to continually monitor the patient's heart rhythm on a cardiac monitor. Function should be assessed together with sensation in view of the risk of damage to deep structures such as tendons and nerves.

Intervention

First Aid

The appropriate first aid for burns is irrigation with copious amounts of cold water. This will retard the process of tissue destruction due to heat and also afford the patient considerable pain relief.

Airway

The first priority for the burns patient is to safeguard the airway, and if assessment reveals problems due to oedema, tracheotomy or intubation will be considered. The A & E nursing team must be able to respond at once to the need for emergency tracheotomy or intubation in such a situation.

Pain Relief

The application of cold soaks (gauze dressing pads and sterile water for irrigation) to the burnt area will usually reduce the pain felt by the patient. The generous administration of Entonox gas will further relieve pain.

In major burns, the administration of intravenous morphine is recommended by many authorities. The best method is to dilute 10 mg of morphine in 10 ml of water for injection, and then to give slowly, sufficient of the drug to achieve the desired degree of sedation and pain relief.

In dealing with young children, sedation is very important as it is impossible to dress properly limbs that are flailing in all directions at once. Furthermore, the more distressed the child, the more distressed will be the parents who are already probably feeling desperately guilty and blaming themselves for their young child's misfortune. A child may be sedated with oral trimeprazine syrup, but it must be remembered that the child can still feel the pain and that therefore some other analgesic agent is required in addition. Wherever possible, when dressing burns on young children, nurses should allow them to sit on their parent's lap as being held by a parent will be a source of comfort in what the child is currently experiencing as a very frightening experience.

Psychological Support

From the nurse's very first encounter with the patient, psychological support will be essential. Reference has already been made to the likely guilt feelings that parents of young children will be feeling. In addition, adults will be fearing disfigurement as a result of their injuries.

It is very difficult at this early stage in A & E to deal with a straight 'Will I be scarred for life?' question. But this is precisely what is in the mind of the burn victim, and may even be on their lips. If asked, the nurse should try to answer the question fairly and frankly, pointing out that at this early stage it is very difficult to say with any degree of certainty what the outcome will be. Such an answer is better than bland reassurances about the wonders of modern plastic surgery. On the other hand, the question may remain unasked; if this is the case, the nurse should try to get the patient to verbalise their fears and to get the matter out in the open for realistic discussion.

The degree of distress displayed by the patient may be markedly reduced by simply talking about the problem and offering support as appropriate.

The IVI and Fluid Balance

If the burn is over 15% of the body surface area, an IVI will be required to prevent hypovolaemia. Apart from nursing assistance in siting the infusion, it will be a key part of the resuscitation effort that an accurate fluid balance be kept. Catheterisation, with hourly urine measurements, is essential due to the risk of renal failure. The kidneys should be able to produce a minimum of 0.5 ml of urine per kg body weight per hour, failure to do so indicates that they are being underperfused and that, therefore, inadequate IV fluids are being given to deal with the burn shock. For an average adult, the hourly urine output should not drop below about 35 ml.

Burns Dressings

The aim of the dressing is to provide an aseptic environment in which, depending on the depth of the burn, either healing can occur or the wound can be readied for successful grafting.

The first step is to debride the wound. Contaminants such as charred clothing and soot should be washed away using copious amounts of sterile water for irrigation. The wound should then be swabbed in antiseptic solution (centrimede and chlorhexidine) and, using a pair of non-toothed McIndoes dissecting forceps, all dead tissue and blisters should be removed. Little pain should be felt by the patient as the tissue is dead; once pain is felt, it is a signal to stop as that tissue is obviously alive!

The wound dressing should be occlusive and secure, in order to preserve the aimed-for aseptic environment, yet at the same time it should be easy to remove for redressing. These criteria are best met with the Flamazine and Melolin dressing technique which consists of spreading Flamazine cream over an appropriate sized sheet of Melolin with a sterile spatula to a thickness of 3–4 mm and then applying this to the burn. The Flamazine will act as a powerful prophylactic agent in preventing infection of the burn, and yet it can also be used for treating infected burns as well; the Melolin will ensure that the dressing is easily removed without sticking.

Because burns will ooze exudate for at least 24 hours, there is a need for a considerable thickness of gauze backing up the Melolin, possibly two large dressing pads thick. The whole dressing should be secured with tape and then by an elasticated tubular bandage rather than crêpe.

Elevation of the burnt limb is essential because of the volume of

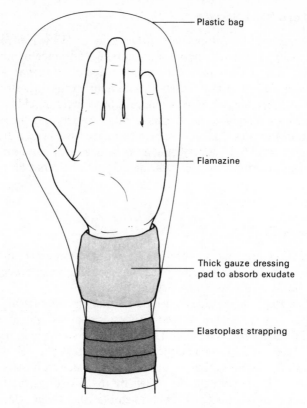

Plastic bag

Flamazine

Thick gauze dressing
pad to absorb exudate

Elastoplast strapping

Fig. 9.3   Flamazine bag treatment for hand burns.

oedema that is to be expected. If the patient is going home, this must be one of the key points made in discharge instructions.

The problems associated with finger stiffness after prolonged immobilisation necessitate the special technique used for burns involving the hands—the 'Flamazine bag dressing' (see Fig. 9.3). Debridement and cleaning are carried out as normal. Then the hand is smeared generously with Flamazine and inserted in a plastic bag which is securely taped to the wrist. A large dressing pad should be taped around the wrist inside the bag to soak up the oedema and the whole arm should be placed in a high arm sling. The key point about this dressing is that the fingers are unrestricted and therefore, providing that the patient remembers to exercise them, stiffness will not be a problem. Instruction about finger exercises is essential prior to discharge.

The same technique may be used for burns to the foot and toes. The nurse will find it a great deal quicker than the traditional burns dressings which would involve separate dressings for each finger in addition to dressings for the rest of the hand.

Self-care of Burns Dressings

The majority of burns patients seen in an A & E department are usually discharged home and followed-up on an out-patient basis. Therefore, the patient must fully understand how to look after the dressing if best results are to be obtained and complications such as infection are to be avoided. Key points are the need to keep the limb elevated in fresh burns, the importance of exercising the fingers in hand burns, and for any burn, the need to keep the dressing clean and dry. The patient needs to know when he or she has to return to hospital—i.e. at an arranged time such as a burns clinic held in A & E, or if the dressing has soaked through, started to disintegrate or emit an unpleasant smell, or if there is another indication of infection.

The ability of the patient or the patient's family to care for the dressing, and the effect that dressing will have on the patient's universal self-care demands should be carefully thought about by the nurse before discharge. Failure to do so can have serious implications for the patient and make for a much more prolonged and painful period of ill health because of the problems that may arise if the burn becomes infected.

Evaluation

The psychological state of the patient, together with the degree of pain being felt, should be closely watched in order to determine the effectiveness of intervention in these two areas. It is also important to check that an elevated limb remains elevated as it may easily slip.

The effectiveness of the other main area of nursing intervention, the dressing, is usually measured at the patient's next attendance. It is important that senior nursing staff check the state dressings are in upon return to ensure that staff within the unit are carrying out effective burns dressings—ie. dressings that will last with a minimum infection rate and which can be easily removed without causing the patient undue distress. It is only by monitoring dressing standards that steps, such as teaching, can be taken to improve dressings to the standard required should there be a shortfall. (See Fig. 9.4 for Standard Care Plan for Burns.)

Date Time	Potential Problem	Patient Goal	Dead-line	Nursing Intervention	Evaluation: Were assessment and intervention carried out as in Nursing Intervention?		
					Yes	No	N/A	Effectiveness in meeting self-care deficit.
				1. Complete Standard Nursing Assessment.			
				2. Obtain data specific to chief complaint:			
				2.1 Area burnt.			
				2.2 Depth of burn (pin prick).			
				2.3 Burn agent.			
				3. Carry out Standard Nursing Intervention.			
	Patient is unable to maintain normal respiration.	a) Patient is to clear and maintain patent airway. b) Patient is to take adequate O_2 into lungs.		See No. 3.			
	Patient feels pain which s/he cannot relieve.	Patient to achieve relief from pain.		See No. 3. 4.1 Assist patient to use Entonox. 4.2 Dress burns with wet soak (where appropriate) 4.3 Administer analgesic drug as prescribed. 4.4 Carry out any special treatment for burn agent.			
	Patient is anxious due to pain/fear of disfigurement.	Patient to reduce anxiety levels.		5.1 Offer support to patient and family.			
	Patient's wound will become infected.	Patient's wound will not become infected.		6.1 Toilet and debride wound. 6.2 Dress wound with Flamazine and non-adherent, aseptic occlusive dressing, maximising function. 6.3 Instruct patient on care of wound/dressing.			

Fig. 9.4.   Standard Care Plan: Burns.

Finally, it remains to check that the information that has been taught has been learnt, i.e. does the patient understand the self-care instructions that have been given? Only questioning of the patient will allow nurses to discover whether he or she has truly learnt what has been taught.

Further Reading

Muir I. F. K., Barclay T. C. (1974). *Burns and Their Treatment.* London: Lloyd-Luke.

Settle J. (1974). *Burns—the First 24 Hours.* Welwyn Garden City. Booklet available from Smith & Nephew.

Wagner M. W. (1977). Emergency Care of the Burned Patient. *American Journal of Nursing.* November. pp. 1788–91.

CHAPTER 10

EYE COMPLAINTS
AND EMERGENCIES

Pathology

The human eye has been well-endowed by nature with defences such as the bony orbit and a very fast blink reflex. Despite these defences, however, eye injuries are common. In addition, the A & E nurse will see many patients who bring themselves to the department with a wide variety of eye complaints of a non-traumatic origin.

The magnitude of the problem may be assessed from the study by Lambah (1968) which showed the ratio of adults to those under 16 years of age suffering eye trauma to be 3:2; Johnston (1971) in a review of penetrating eye injuries showed that the ratio of male to female casualties had changed from 5:1 to 2:1 in a ten year period. Of the patients in Lambah's study, 15.1% were blinded, children faring worse than adults. If just penetrating injuries are considered, it appears that for children 49% of the eyes became blind or were excised, while for adults that figure was 44%. Figure 10.1 shows the principal causes of the accidents.

Non-penetrating eye injury

Trauma to structures surrounding the eye

The bony orbit that surrounds the eye may be fractured as a result of facial or head injury. The injury may be an isolated fracture which is called a 'blow out' fracture or it may be a component of either a facio-maxillary injury or a fractured base of the skull. In a blow out fracture, the cause is a blow to the front of the orbit; the force from the blow is conducted as shock waves by the orbital floor and causes a sudden rise in intra-orbital pressure, the result being that an isolated piece of bone is blown into the adjacent sinus. The problem that this injury causes is that tissue, including muscle, herniates through the hole and becomes

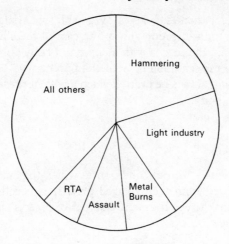

Fig. 10.1 Principal causes of blindness (Lambah 1968).

trapped; the mobility of the eye is restricted and double vision or diplopia develops.

In the more serious cases, where the orbital fracture is part of other fractures, the eye can be impaired by damage to the optic nerve, or one of the other facial nerves, leading to the development of a nerve palsy.

Soft tissue injury to the eyelids is a common situation; it usually causes bruising and usually resolves itself with the passage of time. Due to the speed with which swelling of the lids can develop, it is essential to examine the damaged eye promptly, as soon afterwards, examination may be rendered virtually impossible by the swollen and bruised lids. In burns cases, it may be impossible to close the lids due to the burn damage. As the cornea must not be left exposed (see p. 178), this requires that antibiotic ointment be applied to the cornea and that urgent arrangements be made for a plastic surgery procedure to replace the destroyed tissue.

Foreign body (non-penetrating)

This is probably the most common ophthalmic complaint seen in A & E, the cause being any small particle such as dust, grit, woodsplinters or metal fragments. Foreign bodies which have failed to penetrate the eye will either be found lodged on the surface of the cornea or on the under surface of the eyelid, the conjuctiva. In this latter case, it is known as a sub-tarsal foreign body.

Corneal foreign bodies, such as vegetable material, can produce severe irritation and infection and in the case of metallic objects, can very quickly stain the cornea with a deposit of rust. Sub-tarsal foreign bodies produce the sensation of 'something in my eye' and, therefore, the eyelids should always be everted when a patient presents complaining of a foreign body.

Corneal abrasion

This is an extremely painful condition in which the epithelium of the cornea is removed from the damaged part. It is usually caused by a glancing blow to the eye from any number of objects such as a finger nail, towel or newspaper.

Chemical injury

The extent of the injury is related to the nature and concentration of the agent involved. Alkalis are the most damaging (e.g. substances containing lime such as wet cement) as they can rapidly penetrate the cornea and produce gross damage to the anterior portion of the eye. Acids of equivalent strength are less damaging than alkalis as they combine with tissue components, thereby limiting their penetrative ability. Nevertheless, whether the injury is caused by an acid or alkali chemical, the effects can be devastating.

Radiation injury

Ultra-violet light is the usual culprit, producing damage to the superficial layers of the epithelium of the cornea. Pain, photophobia and watering are the usual symptoms the patient presents with a few hours after exposure. Sun lamps and welding without proper goggles are the usual causes, the latter giving rise to the name of 'arc eye' by which this condition is informally known.

Keratitis or inflammation of the cornea is the usual result of exposure to other forms of radiation. Cataract formation is a long-term complication of ionising radiation exposure. This is well-documented in survivors of the Japanese atom bombs, the cataracts tending to develop some 5 years after the bombing, and in those people who had experienced doses of about 300 rads or more.

Contusion and concussion injury

Contusion refers to injury from the direct impact of the force involved. Damage to the eyelids has already been mentioned; the cornea can also be affected by contusion. The result can vary from corneal oedema through to rupture of the whole globe, depending on the force involved.

Concussion refers to the conduction of shock waves from the point of impact to other parts of the eye. The blow out fracture has already been discussed as an example of this type of injury. Within the globe itself, various very severe injuries are possible, including detachment of the retina or the ciliary body, vitreous or retinal haemorrhages, and /or the development of a hyphaemia. A hyphaemia is bleeding into the anterior chamber and can have devastating effects on sight due to the development of secondary glaucoma and corneal staining. After a total hyphaemia only 36% of patients achieve 6/18 vision. Cataract of the lens or the dislocation of the lens may result from a concussion injury; the iris sphincter may be ruptured in concussion, leading again to the long-term risk of glaucoma.

Penetrating eye injury

Penetrating eye injuries may be classified into two groups: those in which the object responsible is withdrawn after penetration and those in which the object is retained in the eye, forming an intra-ocular foreign body. The prognosis for vision depends upon the size of the laceration in the cornea or sclera, and upon which part of the eye is involved. Penetration to the posterior chamber carries the worst prognosis.

In order that a foreign body may penetrate the eye, it must possess a large amount of energy. Typical objects are glass from a car windscreen, flying debris from industrial processes such as drilling, and material propelled by a blast after an explosion. The most common form of retained foreign body within the eye is metallic—iron and steel account for between 85 and 98% of intra-ocular foreign bodies caused by industrial accidents, a similar proportion to that found in war casualties. Figure 10.2 shows the most common causes of corneal lacerations and intra-ocular foreign bodies. Figure 10.3 shows a patient with a typical car windscreen injury.

A much feared complication of penetrating eye injury is sympathetic ophthalmitis, where after injury to one eye, the uninjured eye develops a severe inflammation some time after (from 3 weeks to 4 months has

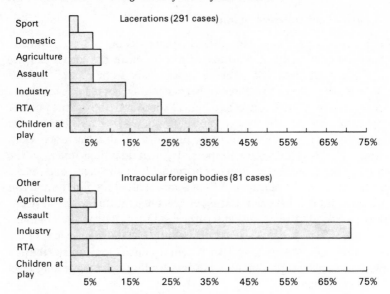

Fig. 10.2 Causes of penetrating eye injury (Johnson 1971).

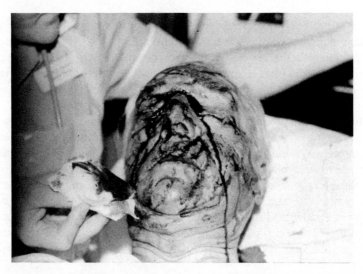

Fig.10.3   Typical car windscreen injury. Serious damage to both eyes plus multiple lacerations to face.

been reported). If untreated, this inflammation leads to loss of useful vision in the uninjured eye in some 50% of cases (Gombos, 1977). Prompt post-traumatic surgery and early enucleation of the injured eye, together with the use of steroid therapy, have greatly reduced the incidence of this complication which can lead to complete blindness.

In addition to the obviously disastrous effects that the foreign body may have on the delicate structures of the eye, there is a further risk of siderosis bulbi if the foreign body contains iron. This condition stems from the chemical reactions which occur within the eye due to the iron, its effects being seen some time after the injury. As the iron dissolves, it becomes incorporated into the cells of the eye, leading to chronic damage and eventually blindness. For this reason, it is mandatory that all ferrous intra-ocular foreign bodies be removed. An electromagnet is commonly used to do this.

Inflammation of the eye

There are many varied eye conditions that bring patients to A & E other than trauma. There is not space to describe all of them, but it is worth noting some of the conditions that give rise to inflammation of the eye, for this is the most common eye problem after trauma.

Table 10.1
Common causes of inflammation of the eye

Condition	Pathology
Stye	Boil on lid margin.
Chalazion	Cyst within tarsal plate (eyelid).
Allergy	Reaction affecting both eyelid and conjunctiva.
Conjunctivitis	Redness of conjunctiva. There is discharge but no pain. Bacteria are the usual cause.
Keratitis	Painful inflammation of cornea. Common causes are an extension of existing conjunctivitis, corneal exposure, or the herpes simplex virus which leads to the formation of a dendritic ulcer.
Iritis	Acute inflammation of the iris.
Glaucoma	Raised intra-ocular pressure. Common cause is blockage of the aqueous circulation from the ciliary body via the pupils to the drainage angle in the anterior chamber. It can be either acute, chronic or secondary to some other condition such as iritis or hyphaemia. This is a potentially blinding condition.

Assessment

The first step is to obtain a history of the complaint from the patient. Important symptoms that may be mentioned and which should alert the nurse to give a patient high priority in the queue include: haloes around lights (classically indicative of an early attack of glaucoma), 'floaters' described by the patient as visible wisps or strands (indicating inflammation or debris from trauma), flashing lights (retinal damage) and, of course, sudden blindness. Other less helpful symptoms (less helpful because they are so non-specific) include photophobia, which may be associated with inflammation of the eye but can be associated with many other illnesses such as migraine and pain in the eye. Pain may be of ocular origin (e.g. inflammation of the cornea), but it may also be caused by many other conditions such as sinusitis, where the patient attributes the pain to the eyeball. Furthermore, the pain of acute glaucoma can be described by some patients as being in the forehead and nowhere near the eyes.

If the patient is presenting with a foreign body, it is essential to find out if it was a high energy or low energy accident, and if possible what the foreign body might be composed of. Similarly, if it is a chemical injury to the eye that the patient has sustained, then nurses need to know what chemical, how long ago and what first aid measures have been taken (hopefully copious irrigation with cold water).

After obtaining a history, the next step is to assess vision. Simple finger counting will assess whether there is any double vision present. The use of the standard Snellen Visual Acuity Test is strongly recommended for all patients with eye complaints. The chart consists of lines of letters of differing sizes which the average eye should be able to read at varying distances, depending on the size of the letters.

The patient is asked to read the chart from a distance of 6 meters, one eye at a time, the other eye being occluded. The results of each eye are carefully recorded, noting the last line to be read correctly. If the patient wears spectacles, this test should be carried out both with and without the spectacles. Each line has a number which refers to the distance at which the average eye should be able to read that line. The result is, therefore, recorded as a fraction, the top number referring to the distance at which the patient stood from the chart, the bottom number being the line number that was correctly read (i.e. the distance at which an average eye would be able to read that line). Thus vision recorded as 6/6 means that at a range of 6 meters the patient can read the same size letters that the average eye can read at 6 meters.

If the patient is illiterate or very young, an E chart is used, consisting of rows of the capital letter E pointing in different directions. The patient is asked to indicate using three fingers the position of the E.

After assessing visual acuity, the nurse should move on to the eye itself, working inwards in a regular sequence which the A & E nurse will find helpful to have as a standard pattern for assessing eyes.

The eye lids should first be examined for evidence of disease or damage. This should include eversion to examine the under surface of the lid (the conjunctiva). This is best done by asking the patient to look downwards, grasping the eyelashes, then gently pulling down, round and up while depressing the upper margin of the tarsal plate with a cotton applicator or similar implement. The under surface of the eyelid should be readily visualised by this technique.

For assessment of the eye itself, a bright pen torch is essential. First the pupil responses and the shape of the pupil should be tested to check they are brisk to respond and equal and regular in size and shape. The cornea should be examined for evidence of a foreign body, a corneal wound or redness indicative of inflammation. Damage to the corneal epithelium is difficult to visualise under normal conditions, but the addition of a drop of sodium fluorescein will show the damaged area in bright green which is easily visible.

Finally, the person as a whole must be assessed. Eye injuries produce great fear of blindness in many patients. Patients are, therefore, likely to be very frightened and anxious. Thus an assessment of the psychological state of the patient is needed as nursing intervention is required in this area as much as for the actual eye injury.

The medical assessment will include a test of the field of vision, a detailed exam using both an ophthalmoscope and a slit lamp. A slit lamp is a binocular microscope with a strong light source that provides a well-illuminated and highly magnified view of the area in question. X-rays will be required if there is a risk of penetrating injury or fractures.

Intervention

The victim of an accident who has suffered serious eye injury will need considerable and immediate psychological support due to the fear of blindness which will probably be uppermost in his or her mind. In the absence of any life-threatening condition, the nurse's first priority should be psychological support. It will be the lot of the nurse to deal with difficult questions such as 'Will my sight be alright?' and 'Am I going to be blind?' from a patient whose face will probably be swathed in bloody bandages. The approach described in the chapter on burns is recommended—i.e. sympathetic, honest and realistic.

If chemicals have been spilt into the eye, copious irrigation with water is the correct first aid procedure. Irrigation will then be continued in A & E, the nurse using a special glass vessel known as an undine to gently trickle saline into the eye, moving from the nasal aspect of the eye, laterally each time. The procedure is best carried out with the patient lying flat and the nurse standing at the patient's head. For effective irrigation to occur, the eyelids must be opened. This will require a great deal of tact and gentleness on the part of the nurse, for most people with an already irritable and possibly painful eye are understandably reluctant to have that eye held open while somebody pours fluid into it. Nurses would do well to try to imagine themselves in the patient's position when deciding how to handle the victim of eye trauma. A kidney dish should be held against the face in order to catch the irrigation fluid and the fluid should not be allowed to soak into the patient's clothes. In the case of an alkali burn (e.g. lime), continual irrigation using one to two litres of saline delivered via an IVI giving set may be required over a period of an hour.

A sub tarsal foreign body can be readily removed with a cotton applicator or a glass rod after eversion of the eyelid. Gentleness and reassurance are required in carrying out the procedure as the patient may find it frightening. Corneal foreign bodies are removed frequently with nothing more than a sterile hypodermic needle, however, the cornea first needs anaesthetising.

Nurses are frequently required to instill various drops and ointments in the patients' eyes. The following table provides information on their uses.

After treatment, consideration should be given to padding the eye. However, eye pads do cause great inconvenience due to the monocular vision they produce (e.g. for drivers) which has significant implications for the patient's self-care demand. They should be used, therefore, only after careful consideration of how the patient will manage with monocular vision. The indication for padding an eye is if there is a defect in the corneal epithelium which will heal more quickly under a closed lid. Instillation of antibiotic ointment and padding may be carried out on a daily basis until healing is complete. The pad is best secured with tape (e.g. Micropore) and a short piece of elasticated tubular bandage. The traditional crêpe bandage method of securing pads is expensive, inconvenient for the patient, time consuming to apply and best forgotten.

In serious conditions such as a hyphaemia or detached retina, rest is

Table 10.2
Eye drops and ointments commonly used in A & E

Type	Examples	Reasons for Use
Local Anaesthetic	Amethocaine Novesine	To relieve pain and allow examination. To allow procedures which involve contact with cornea.
Miotic drops (pupil constricting)	Pilocarpine	To open the drainage angle thereby restoring the aqueous circulation in glaucoma.
Midriatic drops (pupil dilating)	Tropicamide Homatropine	To obtain a clear view of the posterior segment of the eye. Prevent adhesions between the iris and the lens in chemical burns. Patient should not be allowed to drive after use as the focussing mechanism of eye will be disturbed.
Antibiotics	Chloramphenicol Drops 0·5% Ointment 1%	To prevent infection. If both eyes are being treated, two separate tubes should be used and labelled left and right, in order to prevent cross infection. Drops are rapidly diluted and therefore need frequent application (hourly). Ointment will last longer.
Anti-viral	Idoxuridine 0·1% Drops	To treat dendritic ulcers caused by the herpes simplex virus. Requires frequent application.
Stain	Fluorescein	To obtain visualisation of areas of missing corneal epithelium. Green indicates affected areas.
Steroids	Betamethasone	To supress inflammation. Must never be used unless the corneal epithelium is shown to be intact as steroids' supression of the natural defence mechanisms can have disastrous consequences in the presence of herpes simplex.

Date/Time	Potential Problem	Patient Goal	Dead-line	Nursing Intervention	Evaluation: Were assessment and intervention carried out as in Nursing Intervention?		
					Yes	No	N/A, Effectiveness in meeting self-care deficit.
				1. Complete Standard Nursing Assessment.			
				2. Obtain data specific to chief complaint: history, visual acuity, examine lids, conjunctiva, cornea.			
				3. Complete Standard Nursing Intervention.			
	Patient disturbed at fear of blindness.	Patient will reduce anxiety levels.		4. Psychological support. Touch, if both eyes closed.			
	Chemical damage to eye tissue.	To avoid or limit tissue damage.		5. Irrigation with water as first aid, then with saline.			
	Irritation due to foreign body.	Irritation will stop.		6. Removal of FB by irrigation or eversion of eyelid and use of cotton applicator/Assist Doctor as appropriate.			
	Pain due to corneal epithelium damage.	Patient will be able to prevent pain.		7.1 Apply drops/ointment as per medical prescription. 7.2 Apply pad to affected eye. 7.3 Give self-care instruction to patient.			
	Impaired vision after treatment.	Patient will be able to meet self-care demand with impaired vision.		8.1 Teach patient about monocular vision. 8.2 Assess home situation and remaining sight. 8.3 Involve others as required to assist patient meet self-care demand. 8.4 Arrange transport; patient must not drive or ride bike.			

Fig. 10.4 Standard Care Plan: Eye Injury/Disease.

essential as further sudden movements can exacerbate the situation. It is as well, therefore, to have a general rule in A & E that movement should be minimised for patients suffering from any eye injury.

Finally, before discharging a patient home from A & E, nurses must be sure that the patient understands what is required in terms of self-care of their eyes and that they are aware of the correct way to apply the ointment or cream that has been prescribed.

Evaluation

Continual assessment of the patient's psychological status is needed to assess how they are coping with the mental stress caused by the fear of blindness.

After irrigation, the nurse should carefully check the eye to ensure that there is no obvious material present, including by everting the eyelid. The degree of understanding of the patient of self-care requirements should be ascertained before discharge, for it is not what is taught, but what is learnt that counts.

References and Further Reading

Gombos G. M. (1977). *Handbook of Ophthalmologic Emergencies*. New York: Medical Exam. Publishing Co.

Johnston S. (1971). Perforating Eye Injuries, a Five Year Survey. *Trans. Ophth. Soc.*, **91**:895.

Lambah P. (1968). Adult Eye Injuries at Wolverhampton. *Trans. Ophth. Soc.*, **88**:661.

Chapter 11

ENT AND DENTAL EMERGENCIES

The Ear

Trauma

The external part of the ear, the pinna, is composed of cartilage and is commonly involved in injury. It may be lacerated, in which case it may be sutured and treated as any other wound, or it can suffer blunt trauma leading to the formation of a haematoma. In this case, the haematoma can be aspirated under local anaesthesia and a pressure dressing applied, the aim being to prevent the formation of a cauliflower ear.

In severe injuries the whole of the pinna may be cut or torn off, e.g. in a knife fight. In such cases reattachment may be possible, therefore, the wound site should be covered with a saline soak and the missing part retained, preferably dry and in a refrigerator though not frozen.

Foreign bodies in the external auditory meatus are common problems with small children. They vary from beads to live insects in which latter case they should be drowned with olive oil before removal is attempted, as the insects are easier to remove dead than alive. Great skill is required on the part of the nursing staff to gain the cooperation and confidence of the parents and the child. The best approach after explaining to the parents what is going to happen is to sit the child on the parent's lap, wrapped tightly in a blanket so as to keep little hands and arms safely out of the way, and then attempt once to remove the object. If the casualty officer cannot remove it immediately, it is best left and the case referred to an ENT specialist. Further attempts with a struggling child may well lead to the object being pushed further into the ear, risking perforation of the eardrum.

The eardrum is most frequently damaged as a result of a sudden pressure change, e.g. after an explosion or in landing or take-off when flying. A blow to the ear with the hand flat or slightly cupped can produce the same effect. Small perforations will usually heal themselves but large tears may require surgical repair. The usual result of a perforated eardrum is deafness on the affected side.

A common reaction is for people to hit themselves on the side of the head affected or to try to poke something down their ear. Both should be discouraged as they may lead to further damage to the delicate structures of the middle ear. In making disaster plans, it should be taken into account that if an explosion has occurred there may be large numbers of people with perforated eardrums and deafness as a result. It is important to attempt to convey the likely temporary nature of such deafness to people in order to allay anxiety.

Diseases of the Ear

It is probably true to say that in an ideal world people with diseases of the ear would not often be seen in A & E as they should have seen their GP who would have arranged the appropriate ENT specialist referral if needed. A & E departments should not be seen as places to walk into and get a sticky ear syringed on request, and in fact the syringing of ears should not be undertaken in A & E.

A & E staff should not, however, be too dismissive of people with earache for two reasons. First, the ear may be very painful and the patient may be in considerable distress, especially if they cannot get an appointment to see their GP for two days, and second, ear pain may indicate a disease process which could have serious consequences for the patient if untreated.

The usual cause of a painful ear is infection: otitis externa, otitis media (which can be acute or chronic), or mastoiditis. Chronic disease of the middle ear (chronic suppurative otitis media) can lead to complications such as meningitis, brain abscess, and erosion and destruction of bone.

While it may be argued, therefore, that it is an inappropriate use of an A & E department to see patients who have had earache for some time, the nurse nevertheless has a duty to ensure that patients presenting with such a complaint are seen by a member of the medical staff.

One disease involving the ear that can lead patients to attend A & E in a very distressed emergency condition is vertigo. This condition gives rise to an illusion of movement, either that the person is moving, or that the environment is in motion. The cause is a conflict of information from the vestibular sources within the inner ear with information from other sensory systems, or alternatively, when the information supplied by the vestibular system about body movement cannot be coherently assessed by the central nervous system.

Vertigo always produces imbalance, although imbalance is not always caused by vertigo. The person suffering from an attack of vertigo will often fall to the ground and vomiting and nausea are common. The patient will present at A & E collapsed with vomiting. The patient should be laid flat on a trolley with cot sides in place and a vomit bowl available. Acute episodes of vertigo can be very frightening for the patient, therefore considerable psychological support is necessary. An intramuscular injection of prochloperazine (Stemetil) 12.5 mg is often prescribed to help relieve the symptoms.

A common cause of vertigo is Menière's disease, affecting one ear only and most common in onset in people between 30 and 60 years of age. The result is a violent paroxysmal attack, rotary in nature, associated with tinnitus and deafness, which may be one of several attacks clustered together. Migraine is another common cause of vertigo, particularly in adolescent girls.

The Nose

Trauma

Fracture of the nasal bones is the most common facial fracture and is usually due to blunt trauma, e.g. a fall on the face or assault. Deformity which may be obvious at first will quickly be obscured by soft tissue swelling. Reduction should occur before 3 weeks, as fractured nasal bones will set within 3 weeks, but after one week in order to allow the swelling to go down. The need is, therefore, to make an ENT appointment for 7 to 10 days time in order that the ENT specialists can manage the problem thereafter.

Nose Bleeds

There are many reasons for nose bleeds, ranging from trauma or simply blowing the nose too hard in young people through to hypertension and degenerative arterial disease in the elderly. In young people bleeding is usually venous, while in the elderly an area of multiple arterial anastomosis located on the septum, Little's area, is usually the culprit, giving rise to arterial bleeding.

Nose bleeds are potentially very serious, especially in the elderly, and should be carefully assessed by the nurse in the same way that any other serious bleed would be assessed. Blood loss should be assessed by interviewing the patient to find out how long the bleed has been going on, by examining any evidence such as a towel used to try to stop the bleeding, and by asking if the patient has been swallowing any blood as well as spitting it out. Blood pressure and pulse must be measured as hypotension and hypovolaemic shock are possible; an alternative finding is that the patient is hypertensive, and the hypertension has given rise to the nose bleed.

If the patient is hypovolaemic, then the full resuscitation procedure should be activated and should take priority over controlling bleeding in the first stages. Ludman (1981) states that 'An elderly patient who has lost a lot of blood is more likely to die during the next few hours from the effect of loss already sustained than from the results of continued bleeding'.

To try to arrest bleeding, the best procedure is to show the patient how to squeeze the *soft* lower part of the nose tightly. This will control bleeding by compression. Compression should be applied *continuously* for 20 to 30 minutes. The application of ice packs may also be beneficial due to their vasoconstrictor effect. The patient should be sat upright if possible with their head tilted slightly forward and they should be supplied with a bowl and instructed to expectorate any blood that drips into their mouth. The patient should be instructed not to swallow the blood because it will lead to vomiting and also prevent measurement of the blood loss. If direct pressure is controlling bleeding, however, there should be little or no blood dripping down into the mouth.

If the patient is shocked from the bleed, their position should be modified to promote venous return and perfusion of the vital centres by elevating the legs and lying the patient as flat as possible.

We see in nose bleeds a good example of Orem's self-care model of nursing at work, as under nursing guidance the patient meets their own self-care demand in stopping the bleeding.

A spray of Cocaine solution (2.5–10%), a head light and mirror, silver nitrate cauterisation sticks, and a nasal packing set will be required by the medical staff to control the bleeding if direct pressure fails. The medical techniques used in A & E are either cauterisation or nasal packing. The nursing staff must ensure that they know where this essential equipment is kept.

The sight of blood can have a very distressing effect on some people and, young or old, the patient suffering from a nose bleed may need considerable psychological support and encouragement from the nursing staff who should be aware that this is a potentially fatal condition. This is especially true of the situation where the patient is required to compress their own nose for 30 minutes. The temptation to let go soon becomes very great and all the good work done by 10 minutes compression can be undone by 10 seconds curiosity in wanting to see if the bleeding really has stopped.

The Throat

Trauma

Reference has already been made to the need to deal urgently with neck injuries due to the twin threats posed by spinal injury and damage to the soft tissues of the throat which may lead to swelling and airway obstruction.

A common problem encountered in A & E is that of adults who feel they have 'something stuck in their throat', usually a fish or chicken bone. Such objects are usually found at the level of the tonsils or in the upper part of the oesophagus.

In assessing the patient, the nurse should be alerted by the patient describing a sensation of sharp pain on swallowing, especially if it radiates to the ear, difficulty in swallowing saliva, and tenderness over the trachea. Any of these symptoms indicate a real risk of an object being lodged in the throat or upper oesophagus. Unfortunately many such objects are radiotranslucent, e.g. fish bones and many dental plates, but radiography is standard procedure still. If a perforation has occurred, even though the causative object may not show on x-ray, air resulting in the soft tissues will allow the medical staff to make a diagnosis.

The picture is complicated by the fact that a sharp object that is swallowed may well scratch soft tissue, leaving behind a sensation of something sticking in the throat, even though the object has long gone on its way down the alimentary canal. Despite reassurance that there is not a problem and that nothing is stuck, the patient can still feel the sensation of something sticking there, and may not be convinced of the diagnosis. Considerable tact and diplomacy are required sometimes in this situation.

Perforation of the oesophagus or the development of an abscess in the upper respiratory tract due to impaction of a foreign body can have very serious consequences. It is advisable, therefore, to err on the side of caution and most A & E departments refer their patients on to ENT specialists if there is any chance of an impacted foreign body. If the patient is discharged, the nurse should reinforce patient instructions to return if symptoms do not improve or if any feeling of being unwell and feverish, or if pain in the upper chest and neck region, should develop. Mediastinitis developing from a perforation of the oesophagus will make the patient seriously ill, while if a pharyngeal abscess were to develop, there is a risk of occluding the airway.

Hoarseness and Stridor in Children

Stridor in a child with a previously adequate airway is usually caused by infection, but inhaled foreign bodies, trauma from ingesting corrosive agents and allergic oedema are other possible causes.

Croup is caused by acute laryngitis and can be a very frightening experience for both parent and child, a fact that should be remembered by the nurse. Dyspnoea is usually associated with more serious infections of the respiratory tract from the epiglottis downwards, rarely but most seriously epiglottitis. The throat and larynx of such young children in respiratory distress should only be examined by medical staff with considerable experience due to the risk of provoking laryngeal spasm which will lead to a total airway obstruction and cardiac arrest. Tracheotomy in a situation such as this is extremely difficult and the only way of providing an airway may well be by inserting needles into the trachea.

Facial and Dental Emergencies

Facial Trauma

Trauma in the form of a direct blow to the face tends to produce one of several characteristic fracture patterns, which may also involve the base of the skull, leading to CSF leakage (rhinorrhoea from the nose and otorrhoea from the ear).

Blunt trauma to the side of the face is most likely to fracture the cheek or zygoma characteristically in three places, the zygomatic arch, the posterior half of the infra-orbital rim and the frontal zygomatic suture, giving rise to what is known as a tripod or trimalleolar fracture.

High energy trauma affecting the front of the face can lead to fractures of the maxilla. Maxillary fractures tend to follow one of three characteristic patterns, first described by the French pathologist Le Fort (Fig.11.1). A Le Fort II fracture produces very heavy nasal and pharyngeal bleeding which endangers the airway. A Le Fort III fracture commonly involves a CSF leak as there is usually an associated fracture

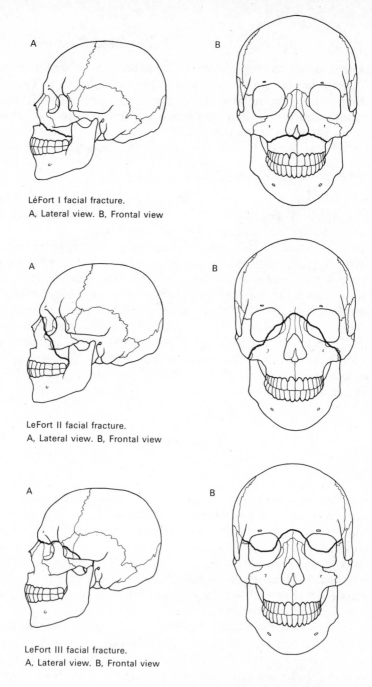

A

B

LéFort I facial fracture.
A, Lateral view. B, Frontal view

A

B

LeFort II facial fracture.
A, Lateral view. B, Frontal view

A

B

LeFort III facial fracture.
A, Lateral view. B, Frontal view

Fig. 11.1   Patterns of fracture, Le Fort Types I–III.

of the cribiform plate. The airway is also at risk in a Le Fort III fracture because, as can be seen, the whole of the front of the face is effectively separated from the rest of the skull.

Fractures involving the mandible are associated with injury to the jaw. A midline fracture will usually be associated with a fracture of the condyles as well. Fractures of the nose have been discussed elsewhere (see p. 184). It remains to add that if blunt trauma affects the eye the result may be a blow out fracture of the orbital floor (see p. 170).

Assessment of Facial Injuries

The first priority in assessing the patient who has sustained facial trauma, as in all cases, is to assess the patency of the airway. Noisy, laboured breathing almost certainly indicates obstruction of the airway. The mouth should be examined for the cause of obstruction, e.g. bleeding, vomit, dentures and the tongue. The contours of the face should be assessed as in a Le Fort III fracture the front of the face is separated from the skull and gives a characteristic 'shoved in' or dish-like appearance. This indicates a serious hazard to the airway due to the abnormal anatomy.

Bleeding should be assessed and its source identified if possible as clots of blood constitute a major airway threat. CSF should be looked for, indicating a fracture of the base of skull if found.

Facial trauma inevitably means that the brain absorbs a substantial amount of the energy involved, leading to the possibility of brain damage. A thorough neurological assessment, with particular attention being paid to level of consciousness, is therefore required.

If the patient is able to cooperate, the ability of the patient to correctly oppose upper and lower sets of teeth should be assessed. Failure to do so indicates facial bone fracture such as a Le Fort or mandibular fracture. Gentle palpation of the face may well allow the nurse to feel the step associated with a fracture. A complaint by the patient of double vision should alert the nurses to the possibility of a blow out fracture causing tethering of the rectus muscle that controls eye movement.

Intervention

The first intervention priority is to clear and maintain the airway which is at hazard from bleeding, clots, dentures, fractured teeth, the tongue, vomit and the abnormal anatomy associated with certain fracture patterns such as a Le Fort III fracture.

The standard measures of mechanically clearing the oropharynx with suction and forceps (or fingers), inserting an oral airway to lift the tongue forward (if tolerated), and positioning the patient on their side with the head down to aid drainage of blood, etc., should be followed immediately. Consideration should also be given to the possibility of cervical injury. In severe cases, intubation or tracheotomy may be required immediately in the A & E resuscitation room. The nurse should therefore know where the necessary equipment is located and be able to give whatever assistance is required by the medical team.

Due to the grave hazard posed to the airway by facial injuries, patients should never be left unattended or lying on their backs. Oxygen may be administered via a high concentration mask. Careful monitoring of the patient's neurological status is required throughout their stay in A & E due to the risk of deterioration in consciousness associated with brain trauma. A cervical collar is a wise precaution due to the risk of spinal injury.

Severe facial injuries can be very distressing to the patient, distress that can be compounded by fear of disfigurement. Psychological support from the nursing staff is therefore very important. Communication with the patient may be impeded as their injuries may interfere with normal speech. Nurses should, therefore, try to phrase questions so that the patient may answer simply yes or no.

Patients with facial fractures will usually have their fractures dealt with by wiring. They therefore need preparing for theatre in the usual way, according to hospital policy.

The effectiveness of nursing intervention needs to be continuously monitored. Evaluation should concentrate on the patency of the patient's airway and also on how much bleeding is occurring, particularly from the nose and mouth where blood can be caught in a bowl and the volume measured.

Dental Problems

It is a regrettable feature of dental practice in the UK that there is no emergency dental service. As a result A & E departments are commonly confronted with patients in severe pain due to toothache for whom there is little we can do apart from give them a bottle of paracetamol.

Bleeding from a tooth socket following an extraction earlier in the day is a familiar complaint seen in the evening at A & E. The presence of blood in the mouth which the patient continually has to expectorate leads to distress and anxiety, while swallowing it will cause nausea and vomiting.

The correct procedure is direct pressure to the bleeding socket applied by having the patient bite on a gauze swab. 'Intraoral bleeders can rarely be clamped and tied and electrocoagulation is of little value' is the verdict of Cosgriff and Anderson (1975), recommending that time and effort should not be wasted on these two techniques.

Usually 20 to 30 minutes of continual pressure will control the bleeding. If this is not successful, the use of an oxidised cellulose dressing should be considered.

It is helpful to ask the patient if there have been any other bleeding-related problems, as this may indicate a significant blood disorder that requires investigation.

Pain associated with facial swelling and an elevated temperature is indicative of a dental abscess, usually related to non-vital or degenerative pulp, the result of advanced dental caries. The patient will often complain of having been unable to eat, drink or sleep because of the condition.

While the medical staff will probably prescribe analgesics and antibiotics (penicillin), the nursing staff should ensure that the patient understands the need for complete rest, which tablets are for pain and which are the antibiotics. This last information should be written on the tablet bottle label as patients who have been suffering from a dental abscess are often tired and distressed and may not absorb fully information given verbally. Dehydration may be present, therefore advice should be given about the need to drink plenty of fluids. General dietary information concerning liquid nutrition may be of assistance in some cases. Such nursing interventions fit well into an Orem self-care model.

In severe cases, cellulitis may develop involving the soft tissue of the whole jaw. Admission for in-patient management is required in such cases.

References and Further Reading

Anderson D. L., Cosgriff J. H. (1975). *The Practice of Emergency Nursing*. Philadelphia: J. B. Lippincott Company.
Ludman H. (1981). *ABC of Ear, Nose and Throat*. London: BMJ.

CHAPTER 12

CHILDREN IN A & E

The needs of children in the A & E department are very different from the needs of adults due to their different physiological, anatomical and psychological development levels. To treat children as no more than little adults is, therefore, a mistake that nurses need to avoid.

Young children are a major component of the case load of an A & E department. A study of 16 000 children born in one week of April in 1970, the National Cohort Study, revealed that by the age of 5, 43% had suffered an accident that required medical attention (Golding, 1983). Ironically, the place that would be expected to be safe, home, is one of the most dangerous to the under-fives. Home accidents accounted for 12% of deaths in the age group 1–4 in one study, while another found that accidents to those aged 0–4 accounted for 23% of all home accidents (Dept. of Trade, 1981).

Parents' perception of danger around the home was studied in an interesting piece of work by Cliff and Li (1983). They found that the three areas rated most dangerous by parents were the kitchen, stairs and bathroom in that order. However, when Cliff and Li looked at where accidents actually do happen, the most dangerous area is the living room, followed by the bedroom and finally the garden. The kitchen, stairs and bathroom were the least dangerous areas in their survey. Of the children involved, 72% of their parents stated that they had had no advice about home safety from a health professional. Based on this study, there is obviously a major role for A & E staff in health education.

Various other social factors are involved in childhood accidents. Of the children in the 1970 national cohort study who died accidentally before the age of 5, 65% of the mothers were in Social Class IV or V or were unmarried. In looking at children who had had two or more accidents requiring medical attention before the age of 5, Golding found the age of the mother to be closely linked—the younger the mother, the more likely the child was to have had two accidents. Children living in rural areas had less risk of accidents than those living in urban areas, so did children whose mothers did not work and interestingly enough, whose mothers did not smoke. This latter finding may be interpreted in terms of the class-relatedness of smoking which shows a heavy bias towards the poorer classes, with more people smoking in the poorer classes than in the better-off classes.

The busy A & E department will see many children, both ill and injured, in the course of a day. It is important that the nursing staff are aware of some of the ways in which children differ from adults, starting with the way that children think.

The way children think and how it varies with age

A child's way of thinking and of perceiving the world is very different from that of an adult. It develops through stages, each of which are very different one from the other. In order that the nurse may communicate effectively with the young child, due recognition of the child's cognitive development has to be made. It is to the work of Jean Piaget and his co-workers that nurses should look for guidance in describing the thought or cognitive processes of a child.

For Piaget, a child has organisations of mental processes called schemata. These are developed by assimilation (the absorbtion and integration of new experiences) and by accommodation (modification of existing schemata). The various stages that a child is described as passing through are:

1. *The Sensori-Motor Stage, Age 0–2.* At this age, the child is said to be egocentric, gradually learning that the world around is not just an extension of self. For the first 7 months of life, the child is without the concept of object permanence; therefore, if something cannot be seen, it does not exist to the child. That something includes both mother and nurse! It is 18 months before the child's actions can be described as purposeful, i.e. the child can work out how to do something before doing it.

2. *Pre-Conceptual Thought, Age 2–4.* Egocentricity is still very pronounced; the child believes that others, including the nurse, think and see the world in the same way that the child does. There is no idea of groups or classes, therefore, the child is unlikely to realise that the nurse who has just appeared is the same sort of person as the nurse who was looking after him or her but who has now gone to lunch. The child cannot deduce as adults can, with the result that if X and Y are alike in some respects, the child may claim that they are alike in all respects. Thus if one medicine tastes nasty, the child may decide that all medicines taste nasty.

3. *Intuitive Thought, Age 4–7*. According to Piaget, it is at this age that the child begins to see things from other people's point of view. But the child is still unable to reverse mental processes with the result that understanding quantity is beyond the child of this age. If liquid is poured from one container into another of different shape, the child will claim that there is more in the container with a higher liquid level and will not be able to see that the volume remains the same. Thus in giving medicine to a reluctant 5 year old, a more successful approach may be to pour the medicine onto a spoon from the measuring pot as the child will think of this as a smaller volume.

4. *Concrete Operational Thought, Age 7–11*. The child develops thought that is defined as logical by adult standards. Reversability and the ability to group and classify are now developed. However, the child cannot deal with abstract concepts, only with those that can be derived from first-hand reality. Thus when a 9 year old Tarzan falls out of a tree and fractures his arm, the instructions to the boy upon discharge should centre upon care of the POP which he can see and understand rather than the healing process of the broken bones which he cannot see and which involves abstract concepts that will not be understood.

5. *Formal Operational Thought, Age 12–14*. It is only in this age range that the child learns to handle the abstract thought patterns and concepts that are taken for granted by adults. However, there are still marked differences between adolescents as they grow into adults in their ability to handle concepts and language codes (see p. 27).

It is true to say that Piaget's ideas and concepts have been challenged by some psychologists. But whatever the final outcome of the academic debates, the nurse should be aware that children of different ages think in different ways, and the nurse should adapt explanations and questions to the child's likely thought processes.

In describing the child's physical development, there are the well-researched milestones which can be summarised by charts such as the Denver Developmental Screening Test. (For this test, see Helberg, 1983.) The use of such detailed screening tests is the role of the health visitor rather than the A & E nurse. However, in assessing young children in A & E, especially in cases of suspected child abuse, it is essential to know what the child should be able to achieve, as underachievement indicates possible understimulation and neglect. Furthermore, in planning A & E facilities for young children, their developmental level is essential knowledge if sensible plans are to be made.

Non-accidental injury

Children whose injuries are non-accidental in origin present to A & E every day of the week. Therefore, it is important for nurses to understand something of the background and the tell-tale signs that should make the nurse suspicious of child abuse—be it physical, mental or sexual. Child abuse is a large-scale problem: Valman (1976) estimates there are as many as 800 fatalities per year from non-accidental injury in the UK, while in the USA, Budassi and Barber (1984) estimate that there are between 50 000 and 70 000 cases per year of which 49% are reported by hospitals, 23% by the police and 12% by schools. The remaining 16% are reported by the parents themselves.

It is dangerous to assume there is such a thing as a typical social setting in which child abuse occurs for it can occur anywhere in the social spectrum—on any street in any town. Dingwall (1983) is critical of the way many professional workers identify non-accidental injury cases for this reason: 'By such means professional staff judge which parents are capable of mistreating their children. In the process they set aside not only middle and upper class parents but also working class families, members of ethnic and religious minorities and mentally incompetent parents. This leaves single mothers and the "rough" working class as most vulnerable to allegations of child mistreatment.' Dingwall's strictures against judging a parent incapable of child abuse by virtue of social class should be borne in mind at all times. In his research, Dingwall did find that nursing staff in A & E units were more alert to and more effective in detecting child abuse than doctors who he criticises for not looking beyond the physical evidence.

In assessing any child in A & E for the risk of non-accidental injury, the following factors should be noted as warning signs:

1. A delay in seeking treatment.
2. If there is an inadequate explanation of the injury.
3. If the explanation is inappropriate for the extent or type of injury.
4. Signs of previous injury, such as fading bruises.
5. Defensiveness and hostility, or alternatively apathy and disinterest towards the child by the parent.
6. Silence and withdrawal on the part of the child.
7. Evidence of failure to thrive; if the child has not reached appropriate milestones both for physical or mental development.
8. Frequent parental attendances at A & E (often for non-specific reasons) with the child.
9. Signs of physical neglect.

If any of the above factors are present, the child should be completely undressed to allow a thorough examination. The behaviour of the child and the parent or parents should be carefully watched as this may reveal clues to abuse that may not be noted if just the physical signs are searched for (Helberg, 1983). Mental cruelty, isolation and neglect of the child's developing mind does not leave physical evidence. Sexual abuse may not either, although the genitalia and rectum should be included in the physical examination. The incidence of sexual abuse of children is difficult to estimate because the better known the person is to the child, the less likely the case is to be reported to the police.

At some stage in the proceedings, the child should be carefully questioned in private, out of earshot of the parents if this is possible. The stage of cognitive development of the child should be considered in phrasing questions. A doll may be helpful in the case of a young child who can demonstrate which parts of their body were interfered with more readily than they can describe with words where sexual abuse is suspected.

Local authorities maintain a register of suspected and at risk children, a copy of which should be in the A & E department, updated frequently, and accessible to all qualified staff. Information that is not accessible is not information. This register should be checked at even the slightest suspicion. Close links with health visitors are essential and the A & E department should liase with the community team at every opportunity.

If there is a strong possibility of non-accidental injury, it is usual procedure to admit the child to hospital, contacting the GP and Social Services at once. The ward staff should be clearly told the likely diagnosis, but the parents must not. Meticulous attention to detail is necessary in recording injuries and marks on the child together with the child's general appearance as the case may well end up in court. If the parents try to remove the child, they must be persuaded not to do so, with if necessary, the final resort of the local Social Services department taking out a Place of Safety Order for the child's protection being implemented.

Cases of non-accidental injury to children can be very distressing for the staff involved. Feelings of anger and outrage at the sight of a pathetic rag doll of a child covered in bruises and burns are understandable human emotions. However, anger is not a constructive force that will help the child. The child is after all the victim of anger. The nurse must be in control of his or herself if he or she is to be in control of the situation and to act for the child in the child's best interests. Remember we are not employed as judges; it is for others to pass judgement on the parents.

Some common childhood emergencies

1. *Accidental Poisoning.* The most at risk age group are those aged 1–4. In 1976 the admission rate was 76·7 per 10 000 in this age group, while for children aged 5–9 the admission rate was only 7·7 per 10 000. For those under one year old, the rate was 22·9 per 10 000. The most common times of day were between 08:00 and 09:00 (17%) and 17:00 and 20:00 (27%), according to a survey by Hancock (1973). Fortunately most of these cases are very trivial as little is swallowed, but the child should be admitted for observation. In 1981, however, 14 deaths were recorded in England and Wales among the under-fives as a result of accidental poisoning.

Substances commonly involved are adult medications (contraceptive pills are commonly ingested), household chemicals (bleach, white spirit, etc.), and wild seeds and berries. In the assessment of the child, nurses need to discover exactly what was taken, how much, when, and if there has been any vomiting since ingestion. Questioning should be tailored to the child's level of cognitive development and also to the mother's level of anxiety which can be very high and as a result interfere with her ability to think clearly.

There are few specific antidotes to ingested poisons; the approach is therefore to attempt to eliminate the substance before further absorbtion can occur. Gastric lavage is to be avoided if possible in children, and instead emesis is induced by giving 15 ml of syrup of ipecacuanha followed by about 200 ml of water which should be flavoured according to the child's taste with cordial. If this does not work, the dose may be repeated. Vomiting is usual within 20–30 minutes. Gastric lavage is only considered if ipecacuanha has failed or if the child's level of consciousness makes vomiting hazardous. If this is the case, for lavage to be safely performed, the airway needs securing by intubation.

If a corrosive substance (e.g., bleach or a hydrocarbon-based chemical such as turpentine) has been swallowed, emesis is to be avoided and drinks of milk given instead. One of the most common and serious poisonings is that due to iron capsules prescribed for the mother's anaemia; they present a very attractive sight to the young toddler. The result is necrosis of the gastrointestinal wall and poisoning by the iron as it is so rapidly absorbed. Desferrioxamine IV should always be available to deal with this serious emergency.

In dealing with the accidentally poisoned child, we should be acutely aware of the mother's distress and guilt feelings. On the other hand, it should not be forgotten that not all childhood poisonings are accidental, a possibility that has to be considered.

2. *Febrile Convulsion.* Children react to illness very quickly, and an acute infection can produce a rapid climb in temperature to over 39°C. As the temperature approaches 40°C, the child becomes very prone to convulsions simply as a reaction to the temperature. Such a convulsion can be a very alarming experience for the parents, who usually wrap their child up in a blanket, increasing the risk of further convulsions by raising the temperature even further, and then rush off to the nearest A & E department in a state of great anxiety.

Great reassurance is necessary, together with an accurate temperature reading (with the thermometer at least 5 minutes in situ, preferably rectally). If the child is indeed pyrexial, then cooling should commence by removal of clothing, blankets etc., and by use of a fan and tepid sponging. The nurse should be explaining to the parents all the time what is being done and why. The source of the infection that is causing the pyrexia should be assessed and treated by the doctor as appropriate.

Epilepsy still has a major stigma attached to it in the minds of many parents, and this thought will be paramount in their minds in many cases. It is best to avoid the word 'fit' and handle the parents with great tact. If the temperature is found to be below 39°C it is unlikely to be a febrile convulsion and some other cause must be considered.

3. *Acute Respiratory Distress.* Pathology: the most common causes of acute respiratory distress in children are:

a. Foreign Body: commonly nuts or beans cause an inflammatory response in addition to obstruction; can be anywhere between the nasopharynx and bronchus.
b. Infectious disease causing obstruction of the airway: a common problem is tonsillitis or a tonsillar abscess. Epiglottitis is a serious emergency as the swollen epiglottis can easily occlude the airway; the child is pyrexial, dysphagic, drooling, hypoventilating but not coughing. No attempt must be made to examine the epiglottis as this can cause spasm and respiratory arrest.
c. Croup: a bacterial infection of the larynx, trachea and bronchi leading to inflammation of the lining of the trachea and larynx. The child is very distressed, exhibits respiratory stridor and has great difficulty breathing.
d. Asthma: the bronchioles are in spasm leading to expiratory wheeze (see p. 95).
e. Bronchiolitis/Pneumonia: the young child can be acutely ill as a result of infection of the lower respiratory tract. Parents may not always contact their GP and can bring such an ill child to A & E at any time of the day or night.

Assessment

A history of the illness should be obtained. The child's respiratory effort and rate need to be recorded together with level of consciousness, colour (if appropriate) and vital signs such as temperature. The amount of understanding of the illness shown by the child and parents needs to be assessed, together with anxiety levels. Examining the airway of a struggling child that is suspected of having inhaled a foreign body is a very hazardous step due to the risk of dislodging the object and causing a total airway obstruction lower down the respiratory tree.

Intervention

Intervention is aimed at both the child and parents. Great gentleness and comfort will be required in handling the child who is likely to be frightened and distressed. As far as possible the parents should be involved with everything that happens. The measures described previously (see p. 62) should be followed, i.e. sitting the child upright, giving high concentration oxygen and carrying out continuous close monitoring of vital signs and respiratory effort. Psychological support for the parents throughout is essential.

Evaluation

Continual monitoring will reveal whether the interventions have been successful in improving the child's respiratory effort. Emergency procedures in the case of a young child in a deteriorating situation are best undertaken by an experienced anaesthetist rather than a Casualty Officer (e.g. intubation, tracheotomy). Fortunately children often respond quickly to the appropriate medication such as nebulised salbutamol, although the doses must be very carefully checked, especially if the A & E department does not receive many children normally.

4. *Sudden Infant Death Syndrome (SIDS)*. Perhaps one of the most tragic scenes of all in A & E is played out several times each day in the UK as an ambulance rushes to hospital with the lifeless body of a young baby and a totally distraught mother who found her apparently healthy baby dead in the cot where she had laid him to rest not long before.

One baby in 500 in the UK will succumb to SIDS. In 1981 there were 1918 male and 1396 female deaths under the age of one year recorded as being due to SIDS. It is a condition that has long been known to humankind, being referred to in such disparate sources as the Old Testament (King Solomon) and the writings of the medieval Welsh priest Geraldus

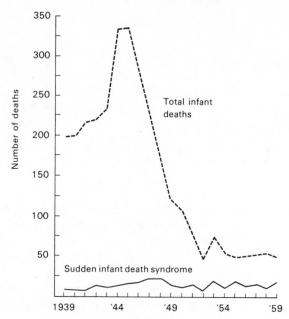

Fig. 12.1 Mortality rate for SIDS, Copenhagen, 1939–1959. While all other causes of infant death have declined, rates of SIDS have remained constant.

Cambrenesis (1188). Despite the dramatic reduction in infant mortality in the last 100 years, the rate of SIDS has remained constant. Figure 12.1 shows how the infant mortality rate fluctuated in Copenhagen during World War II and improved with the rise in living standards after the war; yet SIDS remains stubbornly constant and as a result accounts for a progressively greater proportion of infant deaths.

The age most at risk is 2–4 months and, according to some authorities, in this age range SIDS accounts for more deaths than all other diseases put together. There is a close link with the seasons, the worst death rate being in mid-winter, but by mid-summer this will have fallen to 30–40% of the winter rate. The most common time of day is between 06:00 and 12:00 and the weekend has been found to be the most common time of the week for SIDS to occur.

There is a close link with social class, the poorer classes both in Europe and the USA having the greatest rates (though by no means a monopoly on this tragedy), together with the lowest uptake of post and antenatal care.

However, despite much research and many theories, there is as of yet little real definite insight into the causes of SIDS and hence little that can be done to predict which of any 500 births is the likely SIDS baby. All that can be said is the better the post and antenatal care, the less the risk of SIDS.

Returning to A & E and the nurse confronted with this situation, it has to be said that usually there is nothing that can be done for the infant who is usually beyond resuscitation.

Nurses' attention has to focus on the parents. The nurse will readily appreciate the guilt feelings associated with this situation, especially if the baby has been left with a baby-sitter. It is imperative to try to dissipate this guilt by pointing out that there is no blame to attach and that there is nothing that could have been done. Accidental suffocation is a common idea that springs to the parents' mind in this situation. It is an idea that can be safely dispelled as this is not the cause of SIDS.

The grieving process begins in the resuscitation room and the parents should be encouraged to hold the baby. It is the first step in coming to terms with the reality of death, of accepting rather than denying death, of letting go.

It is essential to arrange support for the family; assistance should be given to contact other members of the family and friends. The health visitor, GP and Coroners Office should be contacted. A post-mortem will be required. Support for the parents may be obtained from the Foundation for the Study of Infant Deaths. Their address is given at the end of the chapter. They are a world famous organisation offering counselling and support through a network of local self-help groups, among their many other activities.

It remains to say that, in addition to the grief of the family, there is also the grief of the staff. Such grief is to be expected as a normal human response to any death, particularly a child's death and staff should therefore be encouraged to verbalise their feelings and emotions. Students in particular find this situation very difficult to handle. In this day and age, there is no place for tears in the sluice and a brusque 'Pull yourself together, girl' from Sister, but rather there should be discussion of the event and support for staff. The dangerous myth of being 'too soft for nursing' should be laid firmly to rest. It is the senior nurses' responsibility to see that such discussion takes place and that staff feelings are thoroughly explored.

References and Further Reading

Budassi S. A., Barber J. (1984). *Emergency Care.* St. Louis: C. V. Mosby.

Cliff K., Li H. (1983). Children in Danger—Community Forum 2. *Nursing Mirror*, 156(7): i–viii.

Dept. of Trade (1981). *The Home Accident Surveillance System; Presentation of 12 months data.* London: Dept. of Trade.

Dingwall R. (1983). Defining Child Mistreatment. *Health Visitor*, 56:249–51.

Golding J. (1983). Accidents in the Under Fives, *Health Visitor*, 56: 293–94.

Hancock B. W. (1973). Accidental Poisoning in Childhood. *British Journal of Clinical Practice*, 3:77.

Helberg J. L. (1983). Documentation in Child Abuse. *American Journal of Nursing*. February. pp. 236–39.

Valman H. B. (1976). *Accident and Emergency Pediatrics.* Oxford: Blackwells.

Note: The address of the Foundation for the Study of Infant Deaths is 5th Floor, 4 Grosvenor Place, London SW1X 7HD, telephone 01–235 1721.

Chapter 13

ELDERLY PEOPLE IN A & E

Just as it is inappropriate to think of children as adults only smaller, so it is wrong to think of the elderly as the same as everyone else only older. The profound physiological, psychological and sociological changes associated with ageing mean that nurses must consider the elderly as having a unique field of problems that is deserving of special consideration.

It is common knowledge that the Western world is in the middle of a population explosion of the elderly. Between 1965 and 1975 the number of people aged 75 or over increased by 16% to reach 5% of the total population, while it was projected that from 1975 to 1985 there would be a further growth of 21% in this age group. The implication is that in the next 10 years, from 1985 to 1995, this 'Edwardian' population bulge will find its way into the 85 plus age group, and an increase of 24% in those aged over 85 is in fact predicted for this period.

Nurses can therefore expect a steady increase in the number of elderly patients coming to A & E departments in the years to come. Apart from emergency conditions that may affect those of younger age (e.g., heart failure, intestinal obstruction), falls are the major cause of the elderly patient being in A & E. It is, therefore, useful to consider the physiological, psychological and sociological changes that occur with ageing and their implications for the care of the elderly in A & E with particular reference to a patient who has suffered a fall. It should be obvious, however, that much of what is said in this context applies whatever the reason for the elderly person being in A & E.

Physiological Changes with Age

There will be a general deterioration of bodily function with age. This is only to be expected, but there are certain key areas which are worth focussing on in some detail, starting with the musculoskeletal system.

There is a loss of muscle bulk and osteoarthritis of various joints leading to pain and stiffness. Such changes seem to affect most old people. In addition there is also thinning of the bone, osteoporosis, which affects females more than males, helping to explain the excess of elderly females who suffer fractures over males, even when the general excess of females in the elderly population is taken into account. Other pathological processes affecting bone become more common in the elderly such as osteomalacia, Paget's disease and bony metastases from malignancy.

The appreciation of pain in the elderly seems much less than in younger age groups. Part of this may be explained by the greater stoicism of the elderly, but it is also thought that there is a real change in the physiology of pain appreciation with age. The absence of complaints about pain should not be taken, therefore, by the A & E nurse as an indication that there is little wrong with the patient. Badly fractured wrists and femurs can elicit hardly a murmur about pain from the elderly person who has had the misfortune to suffer these serious injuries after a fall.

A major problem area is that of temperature regulation which deteriorates with age. Consequently the elderly are very prone to hypothermia even when temperatures are such that a younger person might not consider it cold. A further implication of this loss of temperature control is that many elderly patients do not respond to infection with a rise in temperature as a younger person would. Thermometers are therefore unreliable guides to infection in the elderly, a more likely indication is the sudden onset of confusion, or signs such as a raised respiratory and pulse rate.

The elderly experience many problems with the special senses. Vision deteriorates with age due to changes in the cornea and lens shape that effect focussing, leading most commonly to longsightedness. Diminishing pupillary size and opacification of the lens with old age reduces the amount of light entering the eye to such an extent that a person of 85 needs 8 times as much light to see objects as brightly as a younger person. Problems such as cataracts, chronic glaucoma and retinal detachment all threaten the sight of the elderly. If an elderly person is brought to A & E without a pair of spectacles, the nurse's assumption should not be that their sight is so good that they do not need spectacles, but rather that they have left them behind somewhere in the process of being brought to hospital, and as a result that their vision is considerably impaired.

Hearing impairment increases sharply with age. Degenerative changes in the auditory nerve and cochlea cause a preferential loss of hearing for high frequency sounds, i.e. consonants, which are essential for understanding speech. Problems in sound conduction contribute further to deafness. Many old people therefore rely on lip reading to understand what is being said, and shouting at the patient is of little use except to tell everybody else in the department what is wrong with the patient.

Physical problems do not occur singly in the elderly, but rather there is a multiple pathology. Almost invariably the elderly patient will have several disease processes to deal with at once.

This is a very short summary of some of the areas associated with falls in the elderly, which is why problems such as incontinence have not been referred to. However, in planning care for the elderly in A & E, the nurse needs to take into account all the various physical problems that are relevant to nursing the elderly in any setting. Problems such as pressure areas and incontinence do not go away just because the patient is in A & E.

The Psychology of Ageing

In considering the mental state of the elderly, many nurses will immediately think of confusion as the major problem. Acute confusion is often related to some underlying disease process which once treated will alleviate the confusion (e.g. infection or heart failure). In many cases, however, there is a chronic confusion state. It is thus important to find out upon admission to A & E the person's normal mental state if nurses are to distinguish between a long-standing confusion which indicates either a senile dementia (with histological changes present in the brain) or an arteriosclerotic dementia, and an acute episode.

However, confusion in the elderly may not have a simple physical cause, but may be situational in nature, i.e. it may be the environment and situation that the patient is in that is causing the confusion. It is important to recognise this possibility as simple environmental manipulation by the nurse may control and diminish the patient's confusion without recourse to psychotropic drugs and all their possible side-effects.

In considering situational confusion, nurses should start by looking at the reticular activating system (RAS) which controls the level of activity in the central nervous system. The RAS has an optimum level of sensory input for normal functioning, however, if the input falls below a certain level then a normal level of activation is not projected to the cortex and the organism seeks alternative stimuli in order to function at its normal level.

Experiments show that when sensory input is severely restricted, the effect is to cause emotional and thought disturbance, with visual and auditory hallucinations, and a wide variety of perceptual derangements which are presumably linked to the mechanism described above.

Mitchell (1973) looked at sensory deprivation in relation to nursing and described three situations which make the old particularly prone to suffer from this effect. Mitchell's three types of sensory/perceptual deprivation apply particularly to A & E.

She first talked of a 'therapeutically restricted environment' which corresponds to a typical A & E cubicle: bare walls, no indication of day or night or time of day—an environment totally lacking in stimuli. (Nurses can try lying flat on one of their own trolleys in a cubicle to see how long it takes to get bored.) Mitchell then talks of a 'socially restricted environment' typical of many old people living alone and isolated and also typical of many A & E cubicles where the old person lies for hours, while busy A & E staff go about their work elsewhere. Finally she describes 'sensory-perceptual deficits' associated with the deterioration of the special senses described already and which will be made worse if the patient's spectacles or hearing aid are not available.

So if a patient who cannot hear or see properly is put in an environment with little or no sensory input, the patient will experience severe sensory/perceptual restriction and will be prone to sudden mood changes, thought disorder and hallucinations. Experiments have produced these effects in a matter of a few hours in young volunteers. Therefore nurses may considerably reduce confusion in elderly patients by providing them with an environment rich in stimuli and interaction with other people. A & E nurses should encourage friends/relatives to be with elderly patients at all times. Nurses should try to find time to talk to elderly patients, should arrange cubicles so that there are clues to time and date, should repeatedly tell patients where they are and why they are there (for short term memory characteristically fails with age) and should make every effort to compensate for the elderly patients' failing eyesight and hearing. In short nurses must provide an informative and stimulating sensory environment for elderly people in A & E.

Finally nurses ought to consider the ageing patient as a whole and how he or she views the current situation they are in. Physical limitations on activity can produce frustration; for some people retirement brings hours of empty time and a feeling of worthlessness which results in a fall in self-esteem. Death becomes all too familiar as lifelong friends and relatives succumb to the inevitable passing of the years and this leads to isolation. Anxiety and depression are commonly encountered in old age.

What should be a time of reflection, of looking back at a lifetime and the successful way in which problems were dealt with leading to a feeling of wholeness and integrity, may for others be a time of bitterness and despair, spent contemplating missed opportunities and failures. This in Erikson's view leads to the final life crisis of integrity versus despair, the successful resolution of which is necessary if we are to face death with equanimity and peace of mind.

The Sociology of Ageing

Writing in 1974, Kratz declared that 'Many nurses whether working in hospital or the community take a pessimistic view of old people's families, often implying that they could and should do more for their elderly relatives. This view is understandable though inaccurate.'

A & E departments are regularly confronted with elderly patients who cannot look after themselves but who are not suffering from an injury or medical condition that alone requires admission. As a result A & E staff may fall into the way of thinking described by Kratz, which as she says is inaccurate and may be counterproductive in the long run for the patient.

The traditional view of the extended, pre-industrial family caring for its elderly members in a way not seen today was seriously called into doubt by Laslett (1965) who in a detailed study could find little evidence for such three generation families in the past, and also by the work of Shanas *et al.* (1968).

The modern picture is distorted by two important facts. First, in Victorian times families were on average three times bigger than they are today, therefore the work of caring for elderly relatives was shared out among three times as many people, reducing the individual burden by a factor of three. The second factor is that the previously available reservoir of surplus women whose role was to look after the elderly is now rapidly disappearing as male births exceed female and as women take on different roles in society such as developing a career.

Support for the idea that families care as much for their elderly relatives as they ever did comes from various sources. A study by Isaacs in Glasgow (1971) of the reasons for geriatric admissions found that one-third were with 'therapeutic optimism' in mind, one-third for lack of basic care and one-third due to intolerable strain on the families. Of the group needing basic care due to neglect, virtually all were without families, so family indifference was not the cause. In the third that had families who could no longer cope, the picture was usually one of a family performing heroics over a long period with an elderly relative who was incontinent, disoriented and severely debilitated. From such a picture emerges little evidence of family neglect.

The evidence therefore suggests that the elderly person brought to A & E in a state of neglect will be unlikely to have a family to look after them, while if a family states that they cannot look after granny and she will have to stay in hospital, there are usually good reasons for the family to say so. It is certainly in the patient's best interest not to have conflict between family and hospital, which may easily arise if the A & E staff try to force the issue. After all there are currently close to three million people aged 75 or over in the UK, the vast majority of whom are not in hospital. Who is looking after them? The answer is that families are.

Elderly People Who Fall Over

Having considered some of the physiological, psychological and socio-logical problems that are relevant to the care of the elderly in A & E, this chapter concludes by looking at what is probably the most common reason for the elderly to attend A & E apart from illness, and that is a fall. Much of what is said, however, applies equally well to old people who attend A & E for other reasons.

Problems in mobility caused by joint stiffness, muscle wasting and bone disease are compounded by decay in neuromuscular coordination. The result is that when an old person starts to feel themselves fall, they are unable to adjust their balance as a younger person could to stay on their feet. Hence the much greater frequency of falls in the elderly.

A classic study of falls in the elderly was carried out by Sheldon (1960), and he summarised the causes of almost 500 falls in the elderly as in Table 13.1.

From this series of cases, it appears that one-third of falls among the elderly living at home are from accidental falls, and of the 171 documen-ted, 63 occurred on the stairs while 65 were attributed to slipping or fall-ing over unexpected objects. There is great scope here for accident prevention.

Sheldon's description of a drop attack has attracted much interest. He defined it as a sudden fall to the ground, without warning or any obvious reason (such as a trip) or loss of consciousness. There was usually great difficulty in regaining an upright position afterwards which resulted in many victims being on the ground for several hours. In the study, 58 people suffered the 125 attacks noted, and 26 of them received fractures

Table 13.1
Reasons for falls in the elderly

Accidental falls	171	Tilting head back	20
Drop attacks	125	Postural hypotension	18
Trips	53	Weakness in leg	16
Vertigo	37	Falling out of bed/chair	10
Recognisable CNS lesion	27	Uncertain	23

or dislocations as a result. More recent work has shown drop attacks to be confined to women and to occur almost always when walking, suggesting it to be a peculiarity in the gait of elderly females that causes drop attacks.

Common injuries suffered by the elderly in falls include fractures to the upper end of the femur, wrist (Colles fracture) and upper humerus, dislocation of the shoulder, and lacerations of the shin, scalp and face. Great care has to be exercised with the case of the confused elderly person with a head injury. Is the confusion due to the head injury? The sudden move to hospital in the middle of the night after falling out of bed? Or was the person already confused?

A fracture of the upper end of the femur is a serious injury that most A & E departments see in an elderly person every day on average. The classic clinical sign is shortening and external rotation of the injured leg. A 12 month study of 387 patients with this injury by Pal (1981) could be summarised as follows:

- No seasonal variation in rate.
- Ratio of 4·2 females to each male.
- Most common age group 80–85.
- 54% of fractures involved trochanteric region.
- No bias towards left or right leg.
- 7 day mortality of 3·6%, all due to chest complications.
- Replacement prosthesis performed in 30·6% of cases.

Fractures of the femur require internal operative fixation because the risks associated with the alternative conservative management of 12 weeks or more on bed rest and traction would prove fatal to the majority of elderly persons. Fractures of the wrist are usually reduced and plastered in A & E under regional anaesthesia and followed up on an out patient basis; similarly dislocations of the shoulder are relocated using IV sedation and analgesia. Fractures of the neck of humerus require pain relief and a sling, but can be managed with minimal interference on an out patient basis. Lacerations in elderly people are better steristripped rather than sutured in many cases due to the fragile nature of the skin. This is especially true of flap lacerations over the shins where careful application of steristrips, a non-adherent dressing such as melolin and an elasticated tubular bandage (never crêpe as it always falls down) will produce the best results. On occasions, however, skin grafting is necessary.

Assessing the Elderly Patient in A & E

Assessment should include the psychological and social setting of the patient. Vital information about the state of the person's home can be obtained from the ambulance crew who bring the person to hospital: is it clean, warm and looked after or dirty, cold and neglected? What is the situation with regard to neighbours and family? This and much more key social information is to be gained from the ambulance crew. In undressing the patient, further information may be gleaned about social background by looking at the state of the clothes, skin and general hygiene.

Talking to the patient will enable further information to be gleaned. A first assessment should be made of how oriented the patient is, and of any disabilities due to visual or hearing impairment. Short-term memory should be checked by asking the patient to remember some item and then repeating the question five minutes later. Some elderly people suffer from pathological short-term memory loss yet are able to keep a remarkably good facade of normalcy in conversation, so short-term memory should always be checked. Does the patient know where they are and why? This may seem an obvious question, but nurses will be surprised about how many elderly patients do not—small wonder they are then labelled confused!

In assessing the patient for physical injuries, the principle of multiple pathology should always be borne in mind. Just because there is an obvious fracture of the upper femur, nurses should not forget to look at the wrists and shoulders for possible fractures there also. A full set of vital signs is needed as there may be a whole range of cardiovascular, respiratory, urinary tract, gastrointestinal and endocrine pathologies present as well. Careful temperature recording is essential to eliminate the possibility of hypothermia while the absence of a pyrexia does not exclude an infection (see p. 204). An ECG is fairly standard procedure to eliminate cardiac arrhythmias or a silent MI. Blood sugar should be tested by pin prick and a 'stix' method while urine should also be tested and an MSU obtained if possible.

Intervention—Care for the Elderly in A & E

The dangers of sensory/perceptual deprivation have already been discussed. Every effort must be made to keep the patient oriented in time and space using reality orientation techniques. Provision must be made for the poor memory of the elderly by repeating vital information to them, spectacles and hearing aid should be obtained if at all possible and great care exercised to secure effective communication. Consideration should be given to having a reality orientation board which includes a large clock, the date and a notice of where the patient is. The nurse should remember to use language that the patient will understand.

A & E trolleys are notoriously hard, and pressure sores can have their origins in a long wait in A & E. Turning patients should be as much part of their care in A & E as it is on the wards, however, there is a problem when the patient has a fractured femur as turning would be far too painful. The use of extra mattresses to relieve pressure should be considered. Ripple mattresses are unfortunately too wide for most trolleys but new silicone fibre products are available that are as effective as ripple mattresses in pressure relief and are made in sizes suitable for trolleys. Meanwhile expediting the patient's admission to the ward will help relieve the pressure on their skin and on trolley availability.

The availability of a commode in the department will help many patients for whom perching on a bedpan is very difficult. Small points make a big difference in caring for the elderly. Have they a call button available? The urge to micturate can come suddenly in many elderly patients leading to the humiliation of apparent incontinence, which could have been avoided.

Hypothermia needs to be treated with a space blanket which by virtue of its high reflectivity warms the patient by reflecting their own body heat. The blanket should cover the scalp, from which a very high proportion of heat loss occurs and it should be next to the body. ECG monitoring may be required.

Old people are more likely to accept their lot uncomplainingly, they should not be forgotten therefore in the hustle of a busy A & E department. The offer of a cup of tea while waiting (if they are not waiting for a general anaesthetic) and a few kind words can mean a great deal, and can also obtain for the nurse information that might not have been otherwise volunteered. Elderly people often see real problems as 'something that you just have to put up with', rather than an important symptom.

The problems associated with discharging patients have been discussed elsewhere, however, they are never more pressing than in the case of the elderly. A clear picture of the social background to which we are discharging our elderly patient is necessary before such a step is taken. Given the communication difficulties that arise from declining vision, hearing and short-term memory, it is obviously important to be sure that what has been taught has been learnt with regard to points such as plaster instructions, medication, and follow-up appointments. Simple instruction cards in bold type and medicine bottles that can be opened by the elderly, whose manual dexterity may have declined, are simple examples of planning for the special needs of the elderly.

If care is planned around Orem's self-care model, nurses are more likely to appreciate potential problems from the patient's point of view and, therefore, to make more realistic plans for the patient on discharge. At the end of the day the nurse should not forget her or his role as patient advocate, and if you are unhappy about a medical decision that since the old lady did not break anything when she fell over she must go home, then you must say so. Busy but junior and inexperienced medical staff often overlook the social element of how the patient will cope at home. At the very least, you should ask the doctor to see if the patient can walk unaided, the basic requirement for going home. Many intended discharge decisions have been reversed by such a simple step. Most Casualty Officers are willing to listen to advice from nursing staff about the care of elderly people and their suitability for discharge or about how to get the community services involved provided that the nursing staff go about it in a constructive way.

Evaluation

Evaluation of nurses' attempts to maintain an old person's orientation in time and space is achieved by talking to the patient, and always in language that they will understand. How effective instructions about care of an arm in plaster or about taking medication have been will be seen when the patient next returns—so to some extent we are shutting the stable door after the horse has bolted.

While the patient is in A & E, evaluation can be carried out by checking the condition of the patient at regular intervals to make sure that the trolley is not wet and that pressure points are being relieved.

References and Further Reading

Erikson E. (1963). *Childhood and Society*. New York: Norton.

Isaacs B. (1971). Geriatric Patients: Do Their Families Care? *British Medical Journal*, **4**: 282–86.

Kratz C. (1974). Old People and Their Families. In *The Elderly, a Challenge to Nursing*. London: Nursing Times Publication.

Laslett P. (1965). *The World We Have Lost*. London: Methuen.

Mitchell P. (1973). Sensory Status. In *Concepts Basic to Nursing*. New York: McGraw Hill Book Co.

Shanas E. *et. al.* (1968). *Old People in Three Industrial Societies*. London: Routledge & Kegan Paul.

Sheldon J. H. (1960). On the Natural History of Falls in Old Age. *British Medical Journal*, **2**: 685–90.

Pal A. K. (1980). A Survey of Fractures of the Upper End of the Femur. *A & E News*.

Chapter 14

WOMEN'S HEALTH PROBLEMS IN A & E

by Margaret Judd

A significant number of women who attend A & E do so with complaints that are unique to women. It is essential therefore to explore the background of these conditions in order that the nurse may gain some insight into what is involved in bringing women to A & E.

To understand the present we often have to look at the past, and to understand the origins of many women's health problems, such an approach is essential. In the early 19th century women were a major part of the workforce, having made the transition from their traditional domestic tasks in pre-industrial society to the factories, mills and mines of the new industrial towns. However from 1841 to 1914 they became less and less a part of the workforce as successive Factory Acts limited their hours and pressure from philanthropic reformers and male workers reduced their role in the industrial workforce.

By the beginning of the 20th century, the woman's role was clearly seen to be in the home. This changed briefly with World War I, but when peace returned, women went back from the factories to their domestic duties. Thus in 1921 only 10% of young married women were employed. The provision of 'A home fit for heroes to return to' also included the provision of a job, so those women who had occupied jobs during the war had to leave them.

For some women this proved too much and they insisted that their daughters have an education as good as their sons'. They were to benefit from the 1944 Education Act which provided free secondary education for all and their daughters in turn were to benefit from the expansion in university places that came in the 1960s.

The result of these changes was that by 1971 nearly 50% of married women under the age of 30 were in employment, compared to the 10% of 50 years previously.

Such trends towards emancipation of women and their full participation, as of right, as equals in society have brought many stresses in their wake, related mainly to the dual roles of woman the home provider and woman the worker. It is with these stresses that we will start to consider women's health problems in A & E.

Stress and Women

Many women are now unsure of their place in society as a result of the changes described above. If a woman has children and is able to stay at home and look after them, she may feel guilty as she is not contributing to society. After all, are there not many items in the media telling her how to run a home *and* have a career? However if she does go to work, either out of financial necessity or because she wants a career of her own, she may be criticised for depriving her family of a normal family life (and in times of high unemployment, a man of a job).

In addition, there are many women who are single parents coping with the conflicting feelings described above and all the other problems of being a single parent. In fact only 14% of households consist of the so-called 'norm' of two parents and two children. The 'Janet and John' books in which the mother stays at home all day while the father leaves for work with a briefcase every morning are now a fiction, but the stereotype of that happy family can make the single mother feel inadequate.

There is a strong feeling of guilt when a single mother looks at her children and sees them totally as her responsibility. There is no one to share decisions or control of the children with, no one to help to decide which bills should be paid now and which can wait. It is a great burden to fall on one pair of shoulders.

For both the single and the married woman with children, society creates a situation in which they feel guilty and under considerable stress whether they work or not. Society denies women the right to choose freely between home and work due to the external pressures that are brought to bear on a woman once she has chosen.

In order to give good and appropriate care, A & E nurses should realise the great stress that women have to live with, be they married or single, working or not, as a result of the tensions created by this dual role in society of woman the worker and woman the homemaker.

Some obvious ways that the effects of stress on women have manifested themselves in the last 20 years or so can be seen from statistics on alcohol abuse by women. Between 1964 and 1975, the number of men diagnosed as alcoholics doubled, but the number of women trebled.

Similarly during that decade, the ratio of men to women in mental ill-ness hospitals suffering from alcoholism dropped from 4:1 to 2.5:1. The death rate among women from cirrhosis of the liver, not surprisingly, increased from 25.98 per million in 1970 to 36.27 by 1975. There are many other such statistics which appear to relate increased stress among women with increased alcohol abuse.

Smoking trends provide a similar picture. Of the 16 leading countries in the developed world, 8 reported increases among the numbers of women smokers during the 1970s, but only 3 reported increases in men smokers. Furthermore, 12 of the countries report a downwards trend in male smoking, while only 2 report such a trend for women. The UK stands third in the women's world league table for deaths from lung cancer behind only Hong Kong and Cuba.

The great stresses imposed on women today are further reflected in the figures for self-poisoning. The ratio of women to men who take drug overdoses is between 2 and 3 to 1, depending on age.

Inevitably these stresses bring women to A & E, either because, as they will frankly admit, they just cannot cope, or because the stress causes physical complaints. It is for some a way to rationalise their des-perate desire to have a rest from their responsibilities. Others come to A & E because of an overwhelming tiredness due to the sheer physical strain of life. A & E can be a space to recover from the emotional batter-ing of life that women experience. Convention allows a man to walk out of a house and go down to the pub alone, leaving the children behind, but a woman cannot.

Whether she turns up at the GPs surgery (often as research shows to be dismissed with tranquillisers) or at the A & E department, this woman is not a malingerer nor a time waster, she has a real problem that must be recognised. The nurse should be supportive and sympathetic, not dismissive with a 'Pull yourself together, of course you can cope' attitude. Physical complaints must be accepted and investigated at their face value, even if there is a suspicion that they may be conscious or unconscious rationalisations of the woman's desire for help. Nurses have no right to a judgemental attitude of disbelief in such cases.

The Battered Woman

'One night he came back at 2 a.m. We had an argument and he started hitting me. He jumped on top of me. He laid into me with his fists, with his knees, with his feet. I was bruised all over. My child woke up and came to sit with me. He carried on hitting me and split her lip too. After-wards I started passing blood in my urine.'

This account of the violence that women suffer at the hands of men was given by an Englishwoman at the International Tribunal of Crimes Against Women, 1976. What makes even worse reading, however, is this woman's account of what happened to her when she sought help the following day:

The GP? He gave me a lecture saying that I was breaking my marriage vows if I wanted a divorce.

The Hospital Doctor? He patted me on the shoulder and said that such things occasionally happened.

The Social Worker? Your husband is such a nice man and he is ever so sorry.

Until the 1960s little was heard of the battered wife. That some men beat their wives was known, but it was no one else's business. Since then the matter has come out in the open and there is little doubt that assaults by men against women are disturbingly frequent, as any nurse who has worked in A & E will testify.

Why then do women put up with such treatment? First, they are afraid of even worse violence if their husband finds out that they have talked about it to someone else. Second, there is the defense mechanism of denial—ignore it and it will go away. Then there is the guilt of failure. A woman must be a failure as a wife if her husband beats her, and then she feels guilty at being unable to do anything about the situation for each of the reasons described above. Pictures of the happy family are promoted everyday by the mass media. Not surprisingly, when her own family life fails in a welter of blows and kicks, the woman tries to pre-serve appearances and live up to the happy family image shown in the media.

There is considerable debate about the social distribution of wife beat-ing and there are strong suspicions that it is not confined to the poorer end of the social spectrum. It may just be less well concealed or more openly admitted amongst women from Social Class IV and V back-grounds.

The age at which battering most frequently occurs is more easily de-termined. The National Women's Aid Federation report the most fre-quently battered age group is from 27 to 32 years of age. An NSPCC study of matrimonial violence found the average age of the children involved in such families was 6·33 years. We therefore see a picture where most violence tends to occur in established marriages with young children.

The nurse in A & E must be on the look out for battered women as their problems extend far beyond their immediate injuries. Suspicion should be aroused if the injuries do not tally with the story, especially the classic black eye sustained from falling over. Another factor that is important is pregnancy, for studies show this to be a high risk period for battering, especially towards the end of the pregnancy when the woman finds it very difficult to satisfy the man sexually. Battered women have three times the miscarriage rate of the general population.

It is in the nature of battering to become a chronic problem. A major DHSS study (1980) of 636 women showed that 47% reported that they had been battered for 6 years or more. Such long-term abuse leaves major psychological scars which will be apparent to the astute nurse, e.g. apathy and disinterest. Often the long-term abused woman will recognise that the story she is giving does not fit the injuries, despite which she will still stick to it.

If in this discussion of the factors that should alert the nurse to the possibility of battering, the nurse is reminded of the clues that are looked for in child abuse, then that is no accident. The actors are the same, the scene is the same and the story very similar.

Once the nurse's assessment has suggested battering as the possible cause of a woman's injuries, it is more important than ever to give the patient an opportunity to talk. Privacy is essential and, if an accompanying small child can be entertained elsewhere by another member of staff for a time while wounds are cleaned and dressed, the chances of the woman feeling that she can talk of the major problems she has within her marriage are greatly increased.

In this situation a woman needs time to recover physically and time to think over her situation from a distance; she needs a refuge. Sometimes a friend or family member can help, but this carries a high risk of reprisals from the man as it is relatively easy for him to find his wife's whereabouts.

An alternative is offered by the Women's Refuge Movement and most large towns now have such a refuge. The A & E department should have access via a telephone number to such a safe house, although for obvious security reasons this should be kept as confidential as possible. Many women do not realise that there is an alternative to returning home to the prospect of further beatings.

If children are involved then whatever the outcome of the woman's treatment, even if she opts to return to the home, the A & E department have a clear responsibility to notify the family health visitor. Violence of such force as to put the mother in hospital is highly likely to also include her children as its victims.

Despite counselling about the refuge movement or the offer of help from friends or family, many women still return home to the potential of further violence. The bottom line must be that even if they do, they can still feel able to come to A & E again in the future and be assured of a sympathetic reception, rather than dismissed with an attitude of 'We told you so, serves you right for going back'. Research has shown that women with violent partners tend to leave them and return to them several times, before being able to leave them for good.

Rape and Sexual Assault

'What I felt most strongly was the look in his eyes which completely negated my existence as a human being. I was no longer a person, I was only an object, *his* object.' This description by a rape victim illustrates what many believe to be the true nature of rape—the negation of a human being and her control by another—rather than the narrow legal definition couched in purely physical terms. The desire to control and humiliate that lies behind rape leaves a deep scar on the controlled and humiliated victim. It is important therefore in dealing with the victims of rape that the nurse consider the damage done to the victim's psyche by this invasion of her body and mind, in addition to any obvious physical damage.

The London Rape Crisis Center has shown that in 47% of rapes the assailant was known to the victim. They have also shown that there is no age limit on rape and that the victims can be very young or very old.

With respect to physical care, the victim will have to be examined by a police surgeon and samples taken from various parts of the body such as pubic hair and including a high vaginal swab. The fact that 30% of rapes are accompanied by other forms of sexual abuse and the use of a weapon should alert the nurse to the possible need for swabs to be taken from, for example, the rectum. The aim is to detect seminal fluid, a key factor in assembling a case for the prosecution. To the woman, however, the taking of such swabs, essential as it may be, can recreate the traumas of her ordeal. Therefore, a great deal of psychological support from the nursing staff is required.

After rape many women feel dirty and contaminated and have a great desire to wash themselves. This should be discouraged until after the forensic examination as vital evidence may be destroyed in this way.

The rape victim should not be left alone in A & E, but should be provided with support and attention. This can be most appropriately delivered by a female member of staff. Not only is the victim having to cope with the physical and psychological trauma of what has just happened to her (and this could include serious genital mutilation) but she may also be thinking—how will her husband react? What effect will this have on her future sex life? Do the police believe her story? Do the hospital staff believe it? What will it be like in the witness box where she will be questioned about her usual sexual behaviour and may well feel that she and not the accused rapist is on trial? These and many more doubts combine to press in on the woman to make her feel desperately isolated: do they believe me? Do they think I asked for it by doing what I did? Does it serve me right?

Nurses have no right to be judgemental about their patients and this is no exception to that rule. A feeling of 'She asked for it' is totally inappropriate for the nursing care of the rape victim. No one deserves to be raped. Women should have the freedom to dress as they like and to walk the streets at their will without worrying about this violation.

Trauma and the Pregnant Woman

Pregnancy is a state of normal health. Despite this fact, however, many A & E nurses feel very anxious when confronted by a pregnant woman who has suffered trauma because of the specific ways that trauma can affect the pregnant woman.

Blunt Trauma

a. *Placental separation (abruptio placenta)*. This is the second most common cause of fetal death; maternal death is the most common.
b. *Uterine rupture*. Unfortunately fetal death and hysterectomy is the usual outcome.
c. *Pelvic fractures*. This is the most common serious fracture in pregnant women.
d. *Rupture of liver and spleen*. The gravid uterus acts as a shock absorber and protects many of the abdominal organs from trauma. However, in pregnancy the liver and spleen become distended and displaced making them more vulnerable to injury.

Penetrating trauma

This is usually the result of gunshot or knife wounds and therefore relatively rare in the UK. Nevertheless it is possible given that pregnancy does not exempt a woman from the risk of assault. The gravid uterus protects the woman's abdominal organs very effectively, though at the expense of the fetus.

Premature Labour and Abortion

Trauma may lead to a spontaneous delivery.

Maternal Shock

A woman's blood volume increases by as much as 50% during pregnancy. Serious bleeding with pooling in the abdominal cavity can occur, hidden by the gravid uterus. The increased blood volume of the woman means that she can lose up to a third of that volume, before any signs of hypovolaemic shock appear. The normal response of compensating by shutting down the blood supply to non-vital organs means that the fetus is at great risk in maternal shock, for even in pregnancy, the uterus is non-vital.

Assessment of the Pregnant Woman after Trauma

The usual signs indicating abdominal trauma may be masked or complicated by pregnancy. Stretching of the abdominal wall means that guarding and rigidity are often absent. They are, therefore, unreliable indicators. The increased blood volume associated with pregnancy leads to a situation whereby hypotension and tachycardia may only become apparent when the woman has lost a third of her blood volume.

Any complaint of pain should be taken seriously by the nurse who should ask the patient to describe the pain. Vaginal bleeding is obviously a very significant sign. Fetal heart rate should be monitored in A & E to pick up any signs of fetal distress which indicates the need for an emergency Caesarean delivery.

The psychological state of the woman, together with that of her partner or other friends and relatives should be monitored closely throughout what may be an extremely distressing experience.

Intervention

Resuscitation should proceed along the standard line described earlier, except with the addition of the basic principle that the life of the mother takes precedence over the fetus.

It should be noted that placing the woman in the left lateral position increases the blood pressure and blood flow to the uterus. If the patient is kept too long in the supine position, the effect of the heavy uterus pressing on the vena cava is to exacerbate shock by decreasing venous return to the heart.

Great psychological support is needed for the woman (and her partner if present), both of whom will be extremely anxious for the life of their unborn child. If close to term, the woman may well have dealt with her anxieties concerning the delivery, by reassuring herself that she would deliver in a maternity hospital where they are used to dealing with birth, and where she would be in the hands of a skilled midwife. However, she now finds herself in an A & E department, with staff who have little or no childbirth experience. It is not difficult to see the anxiety that may be produced in the woman as a result.

If a spontaneous delivery does occur in A & E, the nurse can be re-assured by the fact that childbirth is a perfectly normal event that women have been managing to perform successfully throughout the history of humankind. The woman should be allowed to give birth in whatever position she finds most natural and comfortable, which will probably not be on a narrow A & E trolley. If she wishes to squat on the floor, she should be allowed to. The maternity unit should be contacted immediately.

Evaluation

Close continual observation is essential. Vital signs and fetal heart rate must be monitored very closely if the A & E nurse is to accurately evaluate the success of care.

Vaginal Bleeding

Most women between the menarche and the menopause experience vaginal bleeding at approximately monthly intervals. Within that broad statement, what actually happens to individuals varies enormously. For some women a normal period occurs every 3 weeks and lasts 8 days. For others it occurs every 8 weeks and lasts 3 days.

In assessing the patient who attends A & E complaining of vaginal bleeding the nurse needs to discover the following:

1. Date of last menstrual period.
2. Normal frequency and heaviness of periods.

3. Why is this bleeding different?
4. Is there any pain, and if so, its location, type and duration.
5. Is there a possibility of pregnancy?
6. Psychological state of patient.
7. Base line vital signs.

The interview should be conducted in strict privacy, especially if the nurse is dealing with an adolescent/teenager accompanied by her parents. Pregnancy testing equipment should be available in the department.

If the pregnancy test is positive, it is usual to admit the patient to the care of the obstetric or gynaecological medical teams, depending upon the stage of the pregnancy. The patient should be kept still and rested. Any material passed vaginally should be kept for inspection and blood loss estimated from the number of pads used. If the patient is hypovolaemic then urgent resuscitation is required as, for example, a ruptured ectopic pregnancy can cause catastrophic bleeding.

Should the patient have the misfortune to abort in A & E then care must focus on the mother and the loss that she has experienced. The horror of losing her baby may supersede all other thoughts in her mind with the result that well intentioned encouragement, such as 'Think of your other children' or 'There is always another chance', will count for nought. The nurse must recognise that the woman is beginning the grieving process with all that that implies.

Finally the possibility of a criminal abortion should be borne in mind if there are any suspicious circumstances.

Lost Tampons

This is a highly embarrassing but frequent cause of attendance at A & E, caused usually by either a faulty tampon, sexual intercourse during menstruation with the tampon in place, or an attempt to cope with a heavy period by inserting a second tampon. The result of either of these latter two events is to push the tampon high into the vagina where it cannot be retrieved.

Tact and sympathy, a Cusco's speculum, a good light source, and a pair of long-handled forceps will usually permit a female member of the nursing staff to promptly remove the offending article. In order to try to prevent a recurrence of the problem, advice should be offered about the wisdom of sexual intercourse with a tampon in place or of attempting to cope with heavy bleeding by using two tampons.

The Morning After

For some women the dawn brings not only the start of a new day, but the awful realisation of what happened the night before. For a man, finishing the night off with sex is pleasant recreation; for a woman it is pleasant too, but it can spell disaster if she is not taking adequate birth control measures. It is not uncommon, therefore, for women to attend A & E regretting the night before and quite desperate to see if something can be done and asking for 'the morning after pill'.

This is simply a high oestrogen level contraceptive pill that, taken for one or two days and depending upon the manufacturers instructions, will have the effect of inducing a period.

A non-judgemental attitude coupled with advice about adequate contraception are essential. The A & E department should be able to provide a list of Family Planning Clinics and the hours they are open for a woman in this situation for her future well-being.

References and Further Reading

Foley T. S., Davies M. A. (1983). *Rape: Nursing Care of Victims*. St. Louis: C. V. Mosby.

NSPCC (1974). *Yo Yo Children: a study of 23 violent matrimonial cases*. London: NSPCC.

Orr J. (1984). Violence against women. *Nursing Times*, **80(17)**: 34–36.

Pahl J. (1980). *A bridge over troubled waters. Final report on the study presented to the D.H.S.S*. Canterbury: Health Services Research Unit, University of Kent. 1976–1980.

Renvoize J. (1978). *Web of Violence*. London: Routledge & Kegan Paul.

Scott P. D. (1974). Battered wives. *British Journal of Psychiatry*, **125**: 433–41.

The Patient with Behavioural Problems

CHAPTER 15

DELIBERATE SELF-HARM

Patients attending A & E having committed acts of deliberate self-harm (DSH) can be among the most difficult to handle. Their acts represent in many cases outbursts of aggression which have been turned in on themselves or acts calculated to manipulate others. Either way the A & E nurse may find the aggression or manipulation that the patient is displaying focused on him or her.

The ultimate act of DSH is suicide. Over the current century the number of suicides has risen from 3121 in 1901 to 4022 in 1978. However this statement hides many variations, which is only to be expected in such a complex area. The rate for males has declined overall (peaking 1932 with 4045 male suicides) while for females it has dramatically increased, although the current rate is some way below its peak in 1962. The effect has been to halve the male:female ratio for suicides from 3.1:1 in 1901 to 1.6:1 in 1978.

Although current figures represent a higher suicide rate than at the beginning of the century, they nevertheless represent a decline since the beginning of the 1960s. During the period 1963–1970 there was a 32% drop for males and 33% for females. The most likely explanation of this drop is simply the conversion to natural gas with its minimal carbon monoxide content compared to the coal gas used before 1960. However, judging by the last five years, the future seems to indicate an increase in suicide rates again.

One final observation about successful suicides that needs to be made is the finding by Barraclough *et al.* in 1974 that of 100 suicides studied in depth, 90% had some sort of medical assistance within one year of their suicide and 48% within one week. In addition over 80% were receiving psychotropic drugs. These findings indicate that the idea of the 'suicide out of the blue' is not very likely—there are warning signs.

As in all cases of death in A & E, attention should focus on the living. In addition to the devastating effects of a sudden death, the knowledge that it is suicide puts an intolerable strain on the family. The nurse must be aware of this in dealing with relatives of suicide victims as an extra dimension to the grief they experience.

Drug Overdose

If we switch our attention to those patients who do not commit suicide, we immediately are struck by the size of the problem of DSH. Drug overdose is a frequently seen situation in A & E and its incidence has grown spectacularly since the law was changed in 1961 to make attempted suicide no longer a criminal offence. Hospital Inpatient Enquiry statistics for discharges and deaths due to the adverse effects of medicinal agents indicated 23 900 cases in that year; 10 years later (1971), it stood at 85 300 and the rate continued to grow at a slower rate through the decade reaching 106 710 by 1977. The distribution of drug overdose with age and sex is shown in Table 15.1.

Table 15.1
Distribution of drug overdose by age and sex

Age Group	Per Cent	Ratio Female:Male
15–19	16·6	3·26
20–24	18·0	1·85
25–34	27·3	1·54
35–44	17·0	1·75
45–64	15·2	1·67
65–74	3·7	2·00
75+	2·0	1·15

Source: Hospital Inpatient Enquiry 1977

These figures reveal that the problem is worst among the young (61·9% occur in people aged 34 or under), and that females are nearly twice as likely to indulge in DSH than males, and more than three times as likely when they are teenagers.

The statistics so far are only concerned with patients admitted to hospital, but how many present at A & E and are not admitted because they walk out or take their own discharge? (The estimated number of patients presenting at A & E in England and Wales in 1981 was 110 000, of whom 18% were not admitted.)

Table 15.2 shows the variation in overdose rates between different parts of the country. The incidence of overdose is found to be twice as high in the big cities as it is in the country areas, and 50% higher in London and urban areas other than the Metropolitan Areas (e.g. Manchester). This suggests strong links between living conditions, social class and overdose behaviour.

A detailed study into the city of Bristol and environs found the same pattern reproduced on a smaller scale (see Table 15.3) (Walsh, 1982).

Table 15·2
Geographical variation of overdose rates

Area	OD Rate per 10 000 pop.	% ODs discharged from A & E
London	22·8	31·2
Met. Boroughs	30·9	16·9
Urban/Rural	21·8	17·4
Rural	14·7	7·5

Table 15·3
Overdose rates by areas, Bristol and Environs 1980

Area	Pop. age 18 and over	No. of Overdoses	Rate per 1000 Adults
Inner urban	27 842	175	6·29
Council housing	69 695	295	4·23
Flat/bedsits	36 751	113	3·08
Owner occupier	120 402	215	1·79
Dormitory towns	65 390	120	1·84
Rural	44 372	50	1·13

The inner urban area of Bristol contains all the classic ingredients of the rundown inner city. Old housing, much of it in poor condition, blocks of council flats, poverty and unemployment laid the scene for mass rioting in 1980 in what has become known as the St Paul's Riots. The area where the riots occurred has an overdose rate of 14·5 per 1000 adults, more than double the whole of the inner city area.

The council housing consists of large estates on the periphery of the city where unemployment and social problems are high, while the 'flats/bedsits' area is a well-defined area of the city consisting of mostly old houses let off into flats with a high student population.

This study shows the close links between the area where people live, social class, and overdose rates. The stereotype of a bored, middle-class, middle-aged housewife is shown to be, like most stereotypes, inaccurate when considering overdose behaviour.

It remains therefore to ask why do people participate in this form of DSH? In talking to the majority of overdose patients, it quickly becomes apparent that they were not trying to kill themselves. However, within this large number of patients there is a significant number who *are* suicidal, and a trivial overdose may be a 'trial run' before a serious attempt is made. An important task in the nursing assessment is therefore to try to identify those individuals for whom there is a significant risk of suicidal intent.

A frequently found cause of overdose is manipulation of some other person or persons or simply to attract attention. Domestic disputes and relationship problems figure high in the list of reasons, the aim being to bring back a boyfriend or a wife, for example, who has left or is in the process of leaving the overdose patient. Many a reluctant reunion occurs in A & E in the aftermath of a stomach washout. It is frequently the case that the person themselves will raise the alarm, which is consistent with an 'attention seeking' behaviour pattern.

Any behaviour which is rewarded will tend to be repeated. This is a basic guideline in behaviourist psychology, and in it lies the core of the overdose problem. The behaviour of taking the overdose brings rewards, either the person who is being manipulated responds in the way the patient wanted (i.e. comes back) or the attention the patient seeks is provided (ambulances, A & E staff, hospitalisation, visits from friends and relatives). The overdose is a way of coping with a problem and, in the immediate short term, it often succeeds in obtaining the attention or manipulation desired by the patient. The closer the reward is to a behaviour, the more reinforcing it is—another piece of behaviourist theory that is relevant in this situation.

Consideration of the overdose patient's behaviour in this light indicates that there is likely to be a high risk of repeat behaviour. This is indeed the case. When the person next meets a problem or a personal crisis, they are likely to resort to the solution that worked last time and take another overdose, and so a pattern of chronic repeating overdose behaviour becomes established.

One very simplistic assumption to avoid is the sometimes heard opinion that a stomach washout will teach the overdose patient a lesson so that they will not do it again. Such an opinion is wrong on two counts. First, nurses are not in the business of punishing patients—that is immoral and unethical—and second, behaviourist theory shows that the more attention and fuss that is made, the greater the reinforcement and therefore the more likely the person is to repeat the behaviour. If a doctor states that they wish a patient washed out to teach them a lesson, the nurse should refuse to carry out such instructions. If the doctor is so naïve in his or her understanding of human behaviour and wishes to interpret the Hypocratic Oath so as to include punishing patients, then the doctor can do the washout him or herself and take the consequences.

Overdosing can therefore be seen largely as a coping mechanism, aimed at seeking attention or manipulating other persons or situations.

Seen as a problem-solving device, its greater frequency in the poorer areas of towns and cities becomes understandable as people there have more problems and fewer resources to deal with them.

Self-inflicted Injury

Self-mutilation frequently takes a chronic form of repeated episodes of self-laceration usually involving the forearms and varying from the superficial to the occasionally deep. It is rare for there to be any significant arterial damage because the areas attacked are often not adjacent to major arteries in their superficial portions or, in the case of the wrist, the radial and ulnar arteries are well protected by tough tendon sheaths that require considerable force to cut through. Consequently many self-inflicted wounds are easily closed by sutures or steristrips in A & E and blood loss is minimal. Deep structures are rarely damaged, and, if so, it is more likely to be a tendon or nerve than an artery.

Occasionally other areas of the body may be attacked such as the abdomen or legs, while in some very disturbed individuals, the face or genitals may be mutilated. Other forms of self-harm include self-inflicted stab wounds and swallowing objects such as razor blades (usually with the paper still wrapped around them!) or safety pins.

In trying to understand why people behave in this way it has to be recognised that as in cases of overdose, there is usually no suicidal intent but there is certainly a strong streak of low self-esteem in persons who have mutilated themselves. The aggression is often very near the surface, and while it is turned in on themselves in committing the act, the nurse should remember that that aggression could easily be turned outwards if the patient is mishandled.

Assessment

Assessment is broadly similar for acts of DSH whether they be by overdose or self-mutilation.

In approaching the patient to make the assessment, the nurse must remember that the emotional cues given out by the nurse (reflecting his or her attitude) will affect the emotional state of the patient. To minimise the risk of aggressive behaviour and obtain maximum cooperation from the patient, there is a need for a very definite effort on the nurse's part to be friendly and helpful, even though the patient may be hostile, abusive or sullen and withdrawn. An attitude of 'not another overdose' may well rebound back onto the nurse and have an undesirable effect on the patient's emotions and behaviour.

The initial interview should be conducted in privacy. The nurse should aim to find out the extent of the physical damage, and the reasons and intent that lay behind the act. If an overdose has been taken, there is a need to find out what was taken, when, how many and whether the patient has vomited since. If a wound is present, the nurse should examine its depth, type of bleeding (arterial or venous) and assess blood loss and whether any nerves or tendons have been damaged.

Questioning should be sympathetic and carried out in such a way as to allow the patient the maximum opportunity to talk and explain the feelings and emotions behind the act in order that the suicide risk may be assessed. High-risk factors include the presence of alcohol, the absence of close family/friends, the middle to elderly age group, and an existing psychiatric problem which is under treatment (see p. 227). The severity of the overdose is not a reliable guide to suicidal intent. Chronic disease and recent bereavement are further high-risk factors.

If the patient is found to be very drowsy or unresponsive, then a first priority in assessment must be airway patency and other vital signs in addition to attempting to work out what was taken and when. Hypothermia cannot be ruled out if the patient has been lying unconscious for many hours. The vasodilator effect of alcohol would increase this risk and alcohol is found commonly in association with overdose. Rectal temperature measurement is essential. There is a high risk of vomit being inhaled in such cases so that in addition to assessing the patency of the airway, respiratory rate is an important parameter.

Tricyclic antidepressants (e.g. amitryptiline and Anafranil) in overdose have an antiparasympathetic effect which among other effects can cause life-threatening cardiac arrhythmias. A patient who has taken an overdose of tricyclic antidepressants should, therefore, have a 12 lead ECG performed as part of their assessment, and be monitored subsequently.

Throughout the assessment particular attention should be paid to the level of consciousness as a deterioration can endanger the airway. Alcohol greatly increases the effect of drugs such as the benzodiazepines (Valium, etc.) and the barbiturates in decreasing consciousness and may have a significant role to play alone, when the drug taken does not itself produce early impairment in consciousness (e.g. aspirin).

Nursing Intervention

Close and frequent observation is required to monitor vital signs and consciousness, and also to detect any further attempts at self-harm. A

Date Time	Potential Problem	Patient Goal	Dead-line	Nursing Intervention	Evaluation: Were assessment and intervention carried out as in Nursing Intervention?			
					Yes	No	N/A	Effectiveness in meeting self-care deficit.
				1. Complete Standard Nursing Assessment.				
				2. Obtain data specific to chief complaint: 2.1 Substance taken. 2.2 Quantity. 2.3 Time taken. 2.4 Route. 2.5 Sensory abnormalities. 2.6 Breath odour.				
				3. Complete Standard Nursing Intervention.				
	Patient is unable to maintain normal respiration.	Patient is to clear and maintain airway b) Patient is to take adequate amount O₂ into lungs.		See No. 3. See No. 3.				
	Patient will suffer impaired consciousness.	Patient remains conscious. b) Patient will be safe.		4.1 Gastric lavage or give emetic. 4.2 Cot sides or mattress on floor. 4.3 Patient visible at all times.				
	Patient will be hypothermic.	Patient temperature to return to normal.		5.1 Rectal temperatures. 5.2 Space blanket.				
	Patient will suffer sensory disturbance.	Patient will be safe.		6.1 Safety measures as 4.2/4.3. 6.2 Monitor environmental stimuli.				
	Patient will inflict self-harm.	Patient will not inflict further self-harm.		7.1 Observe patient. 7.2 Search, and remove potential implements. 7.3 Offer psychological support.				
	Patient will be depressed and withdrawn.	Patient will be able to talk about overdose.		8.1 Non-judgemental approach. 8.2 Encourage patient to talk.				
	Patient will engage in attention-seeking behaviour.	Patient will end behaviour.		9.1 Do not be provoked. 9.2 Encourage patient to talk. 9.3 Do not reward disruptive behaviour.				

Fig. 15.1 Standard Care Plan: Drug Overdose.

discreet check for potentially harmful items such as razor blades or other tablets should be carried out and any such objects quietly removed.

If there is a chance of recovering undigested drugs or chemicals from the stomach then a stomach washout is performed to prevent their absorption. If this is refused by the patient, a dose of syrup of ipecac (30 ml) should be offered together with several glasses of water to drink; emesis should occur within 30 minutes.

If it is more than 6 hours since ingestion of the drug, there is little point in either course of action as the drug will have passed on into the intestines and been absorbed into the blood. Exceptions to this general rule are the tricyclic antidepressants which because of their parasympathetic blocking effect may stay in the stomach for more than 12 hours, and aspirin which also may be retained in the stomach for more than 12 hours.

If a washout is to be performed, a minimum of two staff are needed. The procedure should be carefully and realistically explained, the nurse mentioning that while it is unpleasant, especially in the passing of the tube during which the patient will experience a gagging sensation, it is not painful and that with the patient's cooperation, the whole procedure can be completed in 5 to 10 minutes. False teeth should be removed, the foot of the trolley elevated to minimise aspiration risk, and the patient positioned on their left side, with a nurse at the head of the trolley with a rigid wide-bore suction catheter (e.g. a Yankaur) ready for use.

The washout tube should be well lubricated with water soluble jelly and passed over the back of the tongue. It will usually fill with gastric contents upon entering the stomach, informing the nurse of its successful placement. The nurse should observe the patient's colour and breathing during insertion as the only other place that a tube that size could go is into the airway, a fact that would be quickly apparent.

A small quantity of lukewarm water should be placed in the funnel at the end of the tube which is then elevated above the level of the patient to allow it to drain under gravity into the patient's stomach. This is then syphoned off by lowering the funnel below the level of the patient. If this first cautious procedure is successful, then the washout should be continued using a funnel full of water each time until the water returning is clear. Encouragement should be given to the patient throughout the procedure. This will help gain cooperation which will make the procedure easier and safer.

If the degree of coma is such that the patient has lost their gag reflex, a washout should only be performed if the patient's airway has been secured by intubation.

Occasionally the patient refuses both ipecac and a washout. It is the patient's right to do so, and while every attempt should be made to make the patient cooperate by persuasion, no attempt should be made by force, and if the patient states that they are leaving the A & E department, they should not be forcibly detained. Only in extreme cases, where there is a real risk to life, is attempting to treat the patient against their wishes justified. In that case, the psychiatric services should be contacted with a view to detaining the patient under a section of the Mental Health Act. If however there is not time to do this, the staff may forcibly detain the patient, but in doing so they must realise that they are committing common assault upon the patient who may subsequently sue for damages under Civil Law. How much damages would be awarded in court against the staff is a matter for contention, as the only precedent for such a case involves the force feeding of a suffragette who was on hunger strike in the early years of this century. In that case, as the prison staff were acting to save the person's life, nominal damages only were awarded. A similar case would obviously be presented in defence of A & E staff forcibly washing out an overdose patient.

Patients who have practiced self-mutilation may attempt further acts while in the department. Physical intervention is not recommended; talking quietly to try to defuse a potentially violent situation is the best way to proceed. The nurse should explain that there is no benefit from such acts and point out that the wounds will be treated appropriately if the patient is willing to allow the staff to help. However, it is very dangerous for the staff and for the patient to engage in a physical struggle as the result may be to accidentally produce a far worse wound than the one that the patient would have inflicted on their own. In addition, the nurse would be rewarding the attention-seeking motivation that lies behind such behaviour in many cases, thereby increasing the likelihood of further episodes of the behaviour.

If the patient is threatening self-harm with a more serious implement than a piece of glass or a razor blade, the best way forward is to talk to the patient and to try to let him or her express their feelings in words rather than in deeds, paying particular attention to what has been said about emotions. Physical intervention is the last resort in such a situation and, if necessary, it should be planned so as to have the maximum degree of surprise and sufficient concentration of force so that the patient is overwhelmed and separated from the implement before they realise what has happened.

The suggested guidelines for handling the patient who has taken an overdose and wishes to leave the department also apply to the person who has committed self-mutilation.

The nursing interventions around those patients who have practised DSH can therefore be seen to be of a conservative, supportive nature —safeguarding the airway, observing closely, offering psychological support where needed, but remembering the high risk of aggression that is present should they turn their self-directed anger outwards, especially as there is usually significant alcohol intake in these cases.

Evaluation

If the patient talks to the nurse about the events that led up to the DSH episode, we may recognise our intervention as being successful, and further self-harm or outbursts of anger are much less likely to occur. The psychological support offered has been effective.

In terms of physical care, the safety of the airway must be checked and evaluated at regular intervals as there can be a rapid deterioration in the level of consciousness. After performing a washout, an estimate should be made of the amount of tablet debris recovered (similarly if the patient has vomited after ipecac administration) in order that the effectiveness of the procedure in removing unabsorbed chemicals from the patient's body may be evaluated.

One final check on the nursing care of patients who have practised DSH is the attitude of the staff towards the next patient who has taken an overdose. If the attitude is one of 'Not another overdose, what a nuisance they are' then the care given is likely to fall short of what is required.

References and Further Reading

For a good general reference, the reader is recommended to read the Office of Health Economics (OHE) publication, *Suicide and Deliberate Self-Harm* (1981).

Walsh M.H. (1982). Patterns of Drug Overdose. *Nursing Times*, **78**: 275–8.

Walsh M.H. (1982). Drug overdose—the national picture. *Nursing Times*, **78**: 1158–1159.

Summary of Drugs Commonly Taken in Overdose
and Actions Required in A & E

Aspirin (Salicylic Acid)

Effect: Metabolic acidosis leads to an increased respiratory rate which may lead to respiratory alkalosis; tinnitus, nausea, vomiting, abdominal pain, sweating, and increased pulse rate.

Washout: Up to 12 hours after ingestion.

Specific Treatment: Forced alkaline diuresis.

Benzodiazepines (e.g. Valium)

Effect: Drowsiness, ventilatory depression.

Washout: Yes, up to 6 hours.

Specific Treatment: Nil.

Paracetamol

Effect: Drug metabolites cause liver necrosis, hepatic failure 5–6 days, death. 20 tablets sufficient to cause severe liver damage.

Washout: Yes.

Specific Treatment: IV Parvolex (acetylcysteine) to limit liver damage if less than 12 hours since poisoning.

Barbiturates

Effect: Metabolic depression, hypothermia, respiratory depression, coma. Potentiated by alcohol.

Washout: Yes, up to 6 hours.

Specific Treatment: Space blanket, watch closely for respiratory arrest.

Paraquat

Effect: Lung necrosis, liver/renal failure. May take several days for effects to appear.

Washout: Yes, up to 6 hours. Leave Fullers earth in stomach after washout to prevent further absorption.

Specific Treatment: Nil.

Distalgesic (Paracetamol and Dextropropoxyphene)

Effect: Dextropropoxyphene is a narcotic and therefore a respiratory depressant; for effects of paracetamol see above.

Washout: Yes, up to 6 hours.

Specific Treatment: Naloxone as narcotic antagonist, see also paracetamol.

Tricyclic Antidepressants

Effect: Blocks parasympathetic nervous system, leading to cardiac arrhythmias, absent bowel sounds, convulsions, ventilatory depression and coma.

Washout: Yes, up to 12 hours.

Specific Treatment: ECG monitor.

Chapter 16

ALCOHOL AND DRUG ABUSE

The nurse will not be long in A & E before realising that alcohol is a major causative factor in attendances, especially at night. In addition, there is now a marked increase in the abuse of various other drugs ranging from solvents to heroin. Effective care planning in A & E requires some background knowledge of who abuses drugs and why and of the social setting within which drug abuse occurs.

Drug abuse may be defined as the use of drugs in an improper or harmful way. The abuser may be addicted, having a physiological need that will manifest itself as the abstinence syndrome on withdrawal, or dependent, having a psychological need to take the drug to cope with life, or neither, being able to take or leave drugs as the whim comes and goes.

Attempts have been made to explain drug abuse in terms of personality types, genetics and physiological factors, but most of these individualistic explanations present serious difficulties. For instance no personality traits have been found that will predict who will become an addict or alcoholic. There are certain traits that have been noted in drug abusers, but these traits have also been found in significant proportions of the population who are not abusers. Furthermore, it is possible to explain such traits as the *result* of the person's drug abuse rather than the cause. Various attempts to establish physiological factors that predispose to alcoholism have failed. Finally, while it is true that having an alcoholic parent considerably increases a person's chances of becoming an alcoholic, no genetic evidence has been found to explain this tendency; on the other hand, social learning theory would strongly suggest that offspring develop alcoholic tendencies by imitating the behaviour patterns of their parents.

A more productive approach to understanding drug abuse is to view it as a social phenomenon. In such a context, we are immediately struck by the fact that one culture will permit one drug as acceptable that another culture will ban. Cannabis and alcohol are obvious examples. Islamic countries ban alcohol but are generally tolerant of cannabis, while the reverse is true in Western countries.

If a drug is readily available within a society, it is more likely to be used. This may seem to be stating the obvious, but it is sometimes overlooked nevertheless. Adolescents therefore abuse solvents because they are readily available. But once they are old enough to buy alcohol, they usually exchange empty crisp packets for empty bottles. The dramatic increase in heroin addiction in the last few years has much to do with the increased availability of the drug on the streets.

Drug abuse may be further understood in terms of peer group pressures. Individuals take drugs because of pressure to conform to a group, or because drug taking is an essential prerequisite for membership of a group.

Once a drug has been tried and found to be pleasurable because of its euphoric or anxiety-reducing properties, or because of the approval of other group members that is gained by the user, then learning theory predicts that this will act as a reinforcer for the behaviour, making its recurrence more likely.

Detailed studies of a wide range of drugs (e.g. Becker, 1953) have shown that the subjective effect of a drug depends very much on the social setting in which it is used, on what the user expects to happen and on previous experiences with the drug. There is a clear analogy with Schachter's work on emotion (see p. 16).

It can be seen therefore that drug abuse is more readily understood in social terms, either on the micro level of groups within society and the pressures and influences that occur at this level and also on the macro level of society itself and how it defines drugs of abuse as opposed to leisure and the availability of drugs within that society.

Alcohol Abuse

The scale of alcohol abuse is difficult to estimate, but one such estimate (BMJ, 1982) talks of 2 million heavy drinkers who run the risk of serious physical damage, 700 000 problem drinkers who are dependent upon alcohol, and 200 000 drinkers who are truly addicted. Given these numbers, it is not hard to see where the estimate of 10 000 deaths a year due to alcohol comes from, together with an estimated cost of £1 billion to the country a year.

The main effect of alcohol is as a depressant, not a stimulant as is commonly thought. Thus in large quantities, it causes drowsiness and diminished level of consciousness, while in moderate amounts removal of inhibitions is experienced. The relevance of this disinhibiting effect to A & E is shown by two studies in Finland carried out by Honkanen (1975). These studies showed that in two hospitals, 86% and 69% of those people involved in fights, assaults and DSH had positive blood alcohols.

In the A & E department, there are two types of alcohol-related problems. First, there is the patient who has some significant other pathology (e.g. a lacerated wrist or a drug overdose) but who is also under the influence of alcohol, and second, there is the person whose problems are solely related to alcohol. This person may be either drunk or an alcoholic who is demanding admission to a psychiatric unit and who may or may not be under the influence of alcohol at the time.

In assessing a patient, whichever of these two categories they fall into, there is a need to ascertain how much they have drunk and how this compares to their normal drinking pattern, how much control they have over their physical and emotional behaviour, and how much insight they have into their present situation. Finally, there is a need to know how long it is since their last drink.

A frequent injury seen in drunk people is severe laceration of the arm from falling on glass. Unfortunately the patient is rarely cooperative enough to permit a thorough examination of the wound, and certainly cannot receive an anaesthetic. In such cases it is best to concentrate on first aid measures to stop the bleeding and if possible to loosely close the wound and wait for morning when the patient will have sobered up enough to be able to go to theatre for proper examination and exploration of the wound with repair of damaged structures as appropriate. If the patient insists on walking out of the department, this should be allowed; they invariably return in the morning with a hangover, but prepared to cooperate in most cases.

Alcohol makes the assessment of head injuries very difficult as one of the key signs is altered consciousness, which could be produced by the alcohol as much as by trauma.

Patients are frequently brought to A & E in a collapsed state due to alcohol intake. In such a situation, their airway must be the first consideration, not only because they may become unable to protect it for themselves, but also because they are highly likely to vomit if they have been drinking heavily. They should be thoroughly examined for other injury, especially head injury. If they are to be kept in the department for some time for observation, it is recommended that they be kept on a mattress on the floor rather than on a trolley. There is less risk of them falling off a mattress and injuring themselves than there is of falling off a trolley.

The effect of moderate to heavy alcohol intake can be to produce aggression. It is important to first of all recognise that it is alcohol that is responsible for aggressive behaviour in an individual rather than other causes such as a psychotic state or a stress reaction, as this will influence the handling of the situation.

Sometimes more sober friends or relatives can be prevailed upon to calm the situation. Whatever happens, the nurse should not respond to shouting or abuse and must keep in control of the situation at all times. Usually the best approach is to enquire politely what the problem is and how the person can be helped; this will often defuse a potentially explosive situation. It is futile to become drawn into an argument with a drunk person as the powers of logic are one of the first casualties of alcohol, and an argument can quickly escalate into violence.

Patients who are alcoholics will occasionally present in A & E asking to see a psychiatrist for 'drying out'. The usual approach of the psychiatric services is that they will only consider a patient for admission if the person is sober and therefore able to exercise clear judgement. If the patient in A & E is under the influence of alcohol, it is unlikely that the psychiatric service will admit them. They are best advised to present to a GP in a sober condition with their request, although if sober in A & E there is no reason why an admission should not be arranged there and then for detoxification and treatment.

At the end of the day, however, despite a 'low profile' approach, it may not prove possible to help a patient under the influence of alcohol, and if they refuse to leave the department when asked, then the solution is to call the police and have the person removed. Nursing staff should not have to act as 'bouncers' in situations such as these.

Narcotics Abuse

The late 1970s and early 1980s have seen a dramatic increase in the supply of heroin to the illegal market in the UK and consequently in the number of addicts. With a 'fix' of heroin now readily available for the price of a cheap bottle of wine, it is hardly surprising that the A & E nurse is encountering an increasing number of narcotics-related problems. These can be divided into three groups: the direct effects of heroin itself, side-effects associated with illegal injection practices, and the abstinence syndrome.

Direct Effects of Heroin Injection

Heroin produces a euphoric feeling. However, like most drugs, it requires a progressively larger dose to produce the same effect as tolerance develops. There is therefore a risk of accidental overdose leading to coma and respiratory arrest.

Furthermore, the heroin bought on the street is impure, having been diluted with additives as the pushers try and increase their share of the profits by making each quantity go further. The result is that what the addict thinks is the normal dose may only be 10% to 30% heroin, with the result that if the addict were to accidentally obtain some pure heroin, there would be an overdose by a factor of many times. Accidental overdose is therefore a common hazard of narcotics abuse.

The overdosed patient will usually be in an unresponsive state, comatose with pin point pupils and severely depressed respirations, if not frank respiratory arrest. A further tell-tale sign that should be looked for is the presence of injection sites or 'track marks', although these need not be present if the patient had inhaled or 'snorted' heroin which is an alternative to injection.

Any patient brought to A & E, aged 20 to 40 years, in a collapsed or comatose state, with no apparent cause, should alert the nurse to the possibility of a narcotics overdose, and the first steps in assessment should be to check the respiratory effort of the patient and the pupil size before looking for evidence of injection sites. Narcotics overdoses outside this range of ages can occur, but they are much less likely.

The immediate aim of intervention is to clear and maintain the airway, and if necessary institute positive pressure ventilation. The patient will need an IV injection of the specific antagonist for the opiate group of drugs, naloxone (usually Narcan 0·4 mg). This will produce a dramatic change in the patient's condition in a matter of minutes, bringing them to a state of consciousness, although they may be a little confused for a few minutes. However, as the half life of naloxone is only an hour, and its peak effect much shorter than that, the respiratory depressant effect of many narcotics is in practice much longer, and the immediate improvement that is observed from naloxone administration may only be transient. It is essential, therefore, that a very close watch be kept on the patient for some time, and several further injections of naloxone may be required depending upon the clinical condition of the patient.

The situation may arise where the patient does not wish to stay for observation. In this case, whoever is with the patient should be informed that the drugs given to counter the effect of the heroin will wear off after a while and the patient may again become comatose. They should be told to keep a close watch and if necessary ring for an ambulance should this occur.

Indirect Effects of Narcotics Injection

The addict who is attending a clinic is sometimes weaned off heroin onto methadone, a synthetic substitute that, although addictive, is taken orally, thereby eliminating the need for injection and producing less disturbance to the daily life of the addict.

However, the street addict will be injecting (as may also the notified addict using methadone), with the result that they frequently attend A & E with abscesses or even septicaemia. The patient may not initially admit to being an addict, however, the nurse should be suspicious of an abscess at an obvious injection site and make enquiries regarding the patient's drug use, reassuring the patient that the police will not be involved and that what is said is in strict confidence (as it should be). The result will often be that the addict will then admit that the true cause of the abscess is an infected injection site.

The importance of establishing a person as an intravenous ('mainline') drug abuser is that the second key risk of illicit drug abuse involving injection is hepatitis B, which is passed on primarily by blood or any other body fluid. It is vital, therefore, that the true status of the addict be discovered in order that the appropriate precautions be taken for everybody's protection, according to hospital procedures and guidelines.

Abstinence Syndrome

The abstinence syndrome, or cold turkey as it is known in the case of heroin addiction, is caused by the withdrawal of the drug after the body has become physiologically dependent upon it. The typical picture in the case of heroin is one of sweating, stomach cramps, vomiting, headaches and tachycardia.

In this situation, the addict is desperate for heroin and may well present in A & E. Extreme caution is required in handling the addict as the desperation can easily lead to violence against members of staff.

Under current legislation and guidelines, however, the prescription of drugs to addicts is strictly limited to certain doctors specialising in the field. It is not, therefore, the place of A & E departments to be prescribing drugs for addicts, no matter how desperate they may appear. Advice should be given about registering with a GP in order to obtain a referral to either a drug treatment centre or to a psychiatrist with an interest in drug addiction. If an addict refuses to leave when refused drugs, the police should be called immediately to deal with the situation. In practice, an addict will usually be able to obtain a 'fix' if turned away from A & E.

An addict's long-term prospects may be assessed by the following results from a long-term follow-up study of 128 notified addicts between 1969 and the end of 1977 (Thorley *et al.*, 1980):

Table 16.1
Long-term prospects of 128 addicts

Attending clinics, maintained on opiates	44%
Totally abstinent	36%
Dead	12%
In prison	4%
Street addicts	4%
	100
Average age at end of follow-up	32·7 years
Average length of addiction	12·8 years

It should be emphasised that these addicts were all attending clinics in the beginning of the study; a follow-up of street addicts would probably reveal even worse mortality and morbidity. However, it should also be noted that of this group, a third were no longer narcotics addicts some seven years later, so the idea of 'once a junky always a junky' does not stand up to analysis.

Hallucinogenics

The effect of these drugs is to produce hallucinations as well as bizarre sensations and feelings, such as being able to hear colours and feel sounds. The best known drug is LSD (lysergic acid diethylamide), although there are other substances such as the so-called magic mushrooms that grow wild in the UK and contain psylocybin as the active ingredient, but whose effects are less potent than LSD. A very powerful agent not found much in the UK is phencyclidine (PCP) or 'Angel Dust'.

The use of LSD has declined considerably since the 'Swinging Sixties' and its associated psychedelia. This is partly as a result of changing fashions and also of a recognition by drug users of the unpredictability and dangers of LSD use. LSD is usually taken in the form of a tablet and usually in a group situation in order that anyone who is on a 'bad trip' may be talked down. However the effects of the drug may be so alarming and disturbing that the users' behaviour constitutes a danger to themselves and possibly others. It is then that the patient ends up in A & E.

The patient's behaviour will often be totally unreasonable and unpredictable as the sensory input will be bizarre and deranged. The need is for a secure environment where the patient may be safely detained without injury, for example, a bare cubicle with a mattress on the floor. If behaviour is disturbed, sedation is required; experience has shown that what is needed is a quick acting IV injection (e.g. diazepam 10 mg) and a long acting IM injection such as chlorpromazine (100–200 mg). Considerable physical restraint may be needed in the first instance to give the IV sedation, and this should only be attempted when there are enough pairs of hands available to do the job safely.

After sedation the patient should be left to sleep off the effects of the drug, under observation, with particular attention being paid to airway and breathing. The patient should also be assessed for injuries that may have been sustained while under the influence of the LSD, as these can be most readily treated at this stage.

Cannabis

Cannabis may be smoked or incorporated into food and eaten. If smoked, its effects appear within minutes. If eaten, it takes approximately one hour to produce its effect. After use, the general feeling is one of mild euphoria and well-being although this is heavily influenced by factors such as the group situation and the users' expectations.

There is little evidence to suggest that smoking cannabis is harmful in the short term, although the occasional patient may present in A & E after their first use of the drug complaining of feeling unwell. It is likely that this feeling is more associated with the anxiety of the individual about the drug experience, than the drug itself. After a short period of observation, such persons can usually be discharged with reassurance.

The toxic effects of cannabis may be gauged from the case quoted by Graham (1977) of a 20 year old male engaged in smuggling concentrated hash oil (an alcoholic solution of the active ingredient in cannabis, THC) by the technique of swallowing condoms full of the oil. One such condom burst in his stomach and, although ill for a day in hospital, he was then discharged with no ill effects. It was estimated that this constituted an overdose of almost 1000 times the normally consumed amount of the drug, nevertheless it did not produce any serious illness. There are very few therapeutic drugs of which the same can be said.

Uppers and Downers

Amphetamines are popular among the younger age group of drug abusers. The feeling of excitement and activity that they produce is greatly increased when they are injected as 'mainline speed'. The user ('speed freak') may go for several days without sleep as a result of IV amphetamine abuse, and be brought to A & E in a collapsed and exhausted condition.

Barbiturates are commonly abused in conjunction with amphetamines, and in addition to all the risks of illicit IV injection discussed under narcotics abuse, there is also the risk of respiratory arrest due to the metabolic depressant effect of barbiturates.

Solvent Abuse

The inhalation of substances for mind-altering reasons has a long history that extends back from the adolescents of today through to the likes of Sir Joseph Priestly, who discovered nitrous oxide in 1776 (N_2O inhalers included Coleridge, Southey and Wedgwood), and back to the Ancient Greeks.

The first solvents to be widely abused were different forms of glue in the USA in the 1960s, the habit spreading to the UK in the 1970s. The substances used are now many and varied, but are mostly based on organic solvents (e.g. toluene, benzene and butane) ranging from glue to nail polish remover, from polystyrene cements to hair spray, and from oven cleaners to petrol. Aerosols are also abused for the effects of the propellants (freons).

A study by Sansum (1984) of a group of solvent abusers referred to a drug treatment centre in the West Midlands found that the mean age was 14, 92% of the group was male, 50% of the group came from broken homes, and although in a multiracial area, none were of Caribbean origins. Her findings are fairly typical of reports from other parts of the country.

The substances are inhaled from a plastic bag (crisp packets are commonly used) held to the face. However, more dangerous practices include placing the bag completely over the head to get a stronger effect (and increasing the risk of death from asphyxiation) and spraying aerosols directly into the mouth which can cause laryngospasm and death.

Mild intoxication is achieved within the first few minutes and can last up to 30 minutes. With careful usage, a user may achieve a high lasting as long as 12 hours. Intoxication is an appropriate word to use in describing the experience felt by many abusers and their behaviour is similar to that of an adult who is drunk. However, there may also be hallucinatory experiences which can lead to extremely dangerous behaviour. Anderson et al. (1982) have identified 117 deaths from solvent abuse between 1970–81, of which 54% were due to the directly toxic effects of the substances used, and 46% to accidents that occurred while the person was under the influence of the drug.

Any adolescent brought to A & E, found collapsed or behaving strangely, should be suspected of being under the influence of inhaled solvents. In assessing the patient, the clues to look for are redness around the mouth and nose, a smell of solvent, the presence of plastic bags/crisp packets in the pockets or the actual substance itself, and changes in behaviour such as an unsteady gait, aggressiveness, slurred speech and inappropriate emotional responses.

The possibility of adolescents in the department sniffing while actually waiting with a friend should also be borne in mind as their behaviour can cause considerable problems. The changes in behaviour described already should be watched for, and frequent visits to the toilet are highly suspicious indeed. The substance involved can usually be smelt on the person concerned.

The aim is to prevent harm to the individual, therefore airway care is the first priority, coupled with detention in a place of safety, if there are hallucinations. Sedation may be necessary. It is important to involve the GP and the boy's family as soon as possible. The family's social worker, if it has one, needs to know as well. Finally, some parents may be unaware that their son is indulging in solvent abuse, so the knowledge should be broken to them tactfully to prevent a hostile rejection of offers of help. Solvent abuse has been found to affect children of all social classes, so the nurse should beware of the trap of falling into stereotyping and overlooking the likely cause of an adolescent's behaviour simply because he appears to be from, for example, an upper-class background.

References and Further Reading

Anderson H. R. *et al.* (1982). Human Toxicology (in press).
Becker H. (1953). Interpreting Drug Experience. *Journal of Health and Social Behaviour*, 8: 166–9.
Black D. (1982). Misuse of Solvents. *Health Trends 1982*, 14: 27–8.
Graham J. D. P. (1977). *Cannabis Now*. Aylesbury: HM + M.
Honkanen R. (1976). *Annol Chirug et Gynaecol*, 65: 282–287.
Paton A. (1982). *Alcohol Problems, Part I*. London: BMJ.
Sansum G. (1984) Glue Sniffing—A Study. *Nursing*, 2 (24): 714–5.
Thorley A. *et al.* (1980). Studying Careers in Drug Dependence. In *Aspects of Alcohol and Drug Dependence* (Madden J. S., Walker R., eds.). London: Pitman Medical.

Chapter 17

THE MENTALLY ILL PATIENT IN A & E

This chapter concentrates largely upon the patient who is suffering from a psychotic condition. Such people are sometimes brought to A & E by friends or relatives and sometimes by the police when bizarre or suicidal behaviour has been acted out in public. Occasionally they wander in off the street themselves. Whatever their mode of presentation, theirs is an emergency condition every bit as much as the person suffering from abdominal pain or having difficulty in breathing.

It is beyond the scope of this chapter to undertake a description of all the various forms that mental illness may take. However, what follows are short descriptions of some of the more common types of mental illness that do present in A & E.

Schizophrenia

Schizophrenia is a profound disorder of thought associated with disturbance of mood, perception and behaviour.

The person's mood is said to be characterised by a poverty of feeling, conversation typically being in a flat monotone with the mood colourless, bland and emotionally dull. There is also said to be an inappropriate affect, i.e. disharmony between what a person says and how they say it.

Perceptual disturbance is associated with hallucinations, usually auditory as the person hears voices telling them what to do next or giving running commentary on events that are happening to the patient. There may be more than one voice audible to the patient. The patient becomes concerned with self, withdrawing from the outside world to live in their own world.

The thought processes become disorganised, illogical and disjointed, leading to the classical thought block where a person stops in mid-sentence, their thoughts having seemingly run into a brick wall. Woolly thinking sometimes characterises schizophrenia; the patient will go 'all the way round the houses' in giving a simple explanation or answering a simple question.

Delusions creep into the patient's thoughts; if these are of the persecutory variety the person will be labelled as a paranoid schizophrenic, one of the traditional four labels attached to schizophrenic patients. (In such a complex area as schizophrenia, it seems very difficult if not impossible to classify patients into one of four varieties of schizophrenia.) Delusions of grandeur are the other common variety of delusional thinking, resulting in a person imagining, for example, that he is Christ or God. Another commonly seen phenomenon is that of ideas of reference where the person thinks there are hidden messages contained in newspapers or TV programmes, for example.

As a result of such profound disorganisation of the mental processes, there is often very bizarre and inappropriate behaviour on the person's part, or they may become withdrawn and inert leading to confusion with depression. Violence may occur in response to what the voices that they hear tell them.

The incidence of schizophrenia is almost one in a hundred, and some two-thirds of patients in mental hospitals are sufferers. The age of onset is typically late teens to early twenties and it can occur in people of any intellectual level or social class.

There are many theories attempting to explain schizophrenia—some genetic, some environmental. Others look for biochemical explanations. It should be noted that there is still another school of thought, typified by Cooper, that denies that schizophrenia exists at all and claims that it is a label hung on people by a medical establishment that is acting on behalf of a repressive society. Cooper's schizophrenics are victims of family disturbance who are reacting in a perfectly understandable way to an abnormal family and social situation. He sees the family as a means of repression of the individual, and the schizophrenic as saying 'No to the mystifying manoeuvres that would forever deprive him of an autonomous existence, separate from the symbiotic obscurities of the family . . . The "No", however, is not heard and the only possibility then is for it to express itself by some other means . . . withdrawal into one's own thoughts so that the words spoken to other people may seem halting, fragmented and disconnected.' Thus Cooper explains thought block and goes on to explain various aspects of schizophrenia as defined by the medical profession (Cooper, 1980).

Depression

Everybody at some time or another has a low in life; for some people though their lows are much deeper than others, so low that all is black and despair and there is no point to life. It is a short step from there to the decision to end life—suicide. Such lows are depression in the psychotic sense of the word.

It is a state characterised by the mood of despair. Associated with this mood are physical changes such as loss of appetite and weight together with inability to sleep; early morning wakening is typical. Some patients will talk of their despair, others will not; there are feelings of helplessness, hopelessness and guilt. Impotence and amenorrhoea are possible.

Mania and Hypomania

The manic individual suffers from excessive elation of mood, irritability, flight of ideas, talkativeness and hyperactivity, all of which combine to produce extreme and bizzarre behaviour. There may also be grandiose or persecutory delusions and auditory hallucinations.

Hypomania may be thought of as a condition where the person's behaviour falls short of the extremes described above, but is broadly similar. It is an easy step to move down the mania scale a little further to the person who is known as the life and soul of the party extrovert. Where does normality end and madness begin? As Cooper has observed: 'Normalization imposes needs rather than recognises them'.

Manic–Depression

It is possible for these two extremes to be combined in the same patient who may function normally for long periods with full insight into their illness, before plunging into deep depression or becoming manic, either way requiring urgent treatment.

Anxiety States and Phobias

Anxiety is a natural feature of life that we all experience, acting often in a beneficial way in motivating us to work hard for an exam because we are anxious that we may fail or in making us careful in crossing the road.

However anxiety can build up for some people to pathological levels, with no apparent cause or focus. Such anxiety is called free floating and may lead to acute panic attacks where the person is convinced that they are seriously ill or about to die. Patients may be brought to A & E in the grips of an acute anxiety attack, exhibiting signs associated with sympathetic nervous system stimulation such as tachycardia, palpitations, sweaty palms and a rapid respiratory rate.

This change in respiration can produce serious biochemical changes due to the lowering in blood CO_2 levels that occurs with overbreathing; this in turn upsets the pH balance making the blood more alkaline which in turn upsets the calcium balance causing muscle spasm (tetany) and tingling in the fingers. There is a characteristic carpopedal spasm of the fingers and abdominal cramps that are associated with hysterical hyperventilation. Their effect is to make the patient even more anxious and therefore more likely to hyperventilate. The solution is to try to calm the patient with reassurance and to try and make them breathe in and out of a paper bag which will have the effect of increasing their CO_2 levels to normal as they rebreathe their own exhaled CO_2. After about 15 minutes, their respiratory rate will be back to normal and the muscle cramps will have abated.

If a person's anxiety is not free floating and instead is attached to some specific object (usually by classical conditioning, see p. 23), then a phobia is said to exist. The most likely phobic state that the A & E nurse may see is agoraphobia—fear of being outdoors—when a phobic patient has a panic attack and is brought to A & E as a result.

Assessment

The nurse will usually be the first point of contact for the patient with the department. Remembering the importance of first impressions, the A & E nurse should greet the patient in a friendly and sympathetic manner. A nursing assessment is required to assign a priority to the patient to see the Casualty Officer, and to decide which is the best environment in which the patient may be looked after within A & E and who are the best persons to be with the patient during this time.

The first step is to sit the patient down in a quiet room with just the receiving nurse present. The offer of a cup of tea may help relax the patient and if he or she wishes to smoke then they should be allowed to do so. Introduce yourself so that the patient knows who you are and that you are trying to help. Try and sit slightly to one side rather than square on to the patient—this is less threatening—and make sure your distance is not so close as to intrude on the personal space of the patient (threatening?) or too far away (disinterested?)—a metre is usually an appropriate distance.

The amount of stimuli in the environment should be kept to a minimum as this may exacerbate the patient's misperception problems or overwhelm somebody who is already feeling overwhelmed by life in general.

Seeking eye contact is an important first step in commencing a therapeutic relationship, followed by a friendly gesture such as the offer of a handshake. The nurse should try to get the patient to talk about their problems, if possible gently keeping them on the subject if they try to wander. It is futile to argue with delusions and hallucinations. This will only provoke anger and aggression in the patient, so the approach should be a noncommittal one, no matter how far-fetched the story told by the patient.

Much vital information that will contribute towards assessment can be gained in these first few minutes by simply looking at the patient. An unkept dishevelled appearance is suggestive of depression or schizophrenia, while bizarre clothing may be associated with mania or schizophrenia. If the person is well dressed and groomed, a full blown psychotic state is less likely, but anxiety neurosis becomes more probable.

Body movements are useful indicators for the observant nurse. Hyperactivity and agitation characterise a manic state while fidgeting, restlessness, facial grimacing and Parkinsonian movements are among the side-effects of the powerful phenothiazine drugs used in the treatment of schizophrenia and, if observed in a person, might give a useful clue to their previous medical history.

Once the nurse has engaged the patient in speech, useful information may be gained from the manner in which the patient talks. A straight refusal to speak suggests withdrawal from the outside world which in turn suggests schizophrenia or depression. A reluctance on the part of the person to initiate speech, which is then slow and hesitant is associated with depression. Not surprisingly, the opposite situation, an uninterruptable flood of speech, is associated with manic states.

The content of the person's speech will tell us much about their thought processes. Schizophrenia is characterised by disordered thought and this is reflected in the speech of the person, it being vague, woolly and halting and incorporating looseness of association, e.g. if the patient is a virgin, so is the Virgin Mary, therefore the patient is the Virgin Mary. Thought block manifests itself by the patient stopping suddenly in the middle of a sentence, their mind a blank—in the midst of thought, there is no thought. The chaotic state of their thoughts leads the person to move randomly between unconnected statements. In addition, the person will describe delusions and hallucinations, and may be seen conversing with the voices that they can hear inside their head.

The person with great pressure of speech, leaping from idea to idea, is exhibiting all the traits of mania. This is known as 'flight of ideas', while the person who remains fixed on one topic is displaying obsession associated with neurosis and anxiety. Expressions of hopelessness, worthlessness or guilt are associated with depression, as has been mentioned already.

The patient's mood should be assessed in this preliminary interview. Whether the mood fits with the ideas being expressed by the patient should also be assessed, as in schizophrenia classically it does not.

Orientation in time and space should be assessed together with how much insight the person has into their illness. If the person does not think they are ill, they are unlikely to want to go to hospital, and there is nothing mad about that.

It remains to try and find out something of the person's life history— where they are from, whether they have been ill before, what their family background is, and so on. Some persons may be known to the local psychiatric service already, others may be presenting with illness for the first time, while others may have come from afar, which should make the nurse alert to the possibility of psychiatric Munchhausen's syndrome (see p. 265).

After the initial assessment, the person's family should be interviewed also if they are present, and they should be involved in the person's care throughout their stay in the department, providing that meets with the approval of the patient.

During the assessment, the nurse should also consider the possibility that the patient's behaviour may be due to drugs. This possibility should be raised with the patient and evidence of drug taking should be looked for. Solvent abuse, LSD, psylocybin and alcohol withdrawal (delirium tremens) can all lead to hallucinations. An adolescent male brought to A & E because of bizarre behaviour is more likely to be under the influence of solvents than suffering from any psychotic state.

It is not the purpose of this initial interview to arrive at a psychiatric diagnosis (which the psychiatrists themselves may not be able to do after several weeks in hospital), but rather to assess if the patient is showing signs that are likely to be associated with an acute psychotic state and to assign a priority for the Casualty Officer to see this patient.

In prioritising the patient, the nurse should remember that acute psychotic conditions do not lend themselves to waiting for lengthy periods—the patient may abscond, cause serious disruption to the running of the department, or inflict serious harm on themselves.

Intervention

The safety of the patient and the staff are the paramount concerns. There should be a quiet, separate room, with minimal stimulation where the patient may be kept. This room should be carefully furnished to avoid providing ready-made ammunition to a very disturbed patient and should have windows that cannot be opened fully so that the patient cannot leave or attempt to leave via that route. Continual observation of the room from outside should be possible, and the patient should not be left alone at any period. If the family are not able to stay with the patient, a nurse should be assigned to this task, and as far as possible the same nurse should stay with the patient throughout their stay in the department, in order to give a feeling of security and to try to build up some sort of relationship.

After the patient has been seen by the medical staff, admission may be arranged to a psychiatric bed. The A & E department is, therefore, assessing the patient and carrying out a holding action until admission can be arranged and therapy commenced. Should violence look likely, the nurse should act in accordance with the principles laid down on p. 268.

Many people arrive at A & E departments in an acutely disturbed state, noisy and behaving in a very bizarre fashion, but leave quietly an hour or so later for a psychiatric hospital and treatment, simply because the nursing staff sat and talked with the patient, in between medical assessments. Force or drugs are not used, the secret being simply to let the patient talk and say what they want to say. The nurse need neither agree (and thereby collude with the patient's delusions) nor disagree (and provoke aggression), but simply allow the patient the opportunity of self-expression. It is worth considering that patients today who are labelled as schizophrenics would in another time and place have been hailed as great prophets and holy people due to their visions and ability to hear God talking to them.

In concluding the chapter we need to look at the situation in which the patient will not cooperate, and treatment/detention in hospital against the patient's will is called for. This requires invoking a section of the Mental Health Act (1983), and Table 17.1 summarises the sections of the Act most likely to be used in A & E.

As can be seen from a study of Table 17.1, the A & E department may receive patients brought by a member of the police force, under section 136, due to their behaviour in a public place. Alternatively departments may receive a patient whose physical health requires treatment before their mental health, under section 135. Such patients are usually elderly and living alone, suffering from malnutrition, hypothermia and gross neglect.

The other section of the Act most likely to be applied is section 4, where the patient is in A & E and the decision is taken that for their own protection and well-being they must be taken into psychiatric care against their will. However patients may also attend A & E from a psychiatric hospital, who are detained under section 2 or 3 already, due to injuries or illness.

Part IV of the Act establishes several categories of treatment, each with specific legal safeguards, which can be administered to certain patients without their consent, e.g. ECT or drug therapy. Part IV does not apply to various types of patients, including all involuntary patients and those detained for 72 hours or less. Before treating a patient, therefore, the A & E department needs consent, which if withheld by the patient, means that the department should check carefully with psychiatric colleagues that it is permitted to administer treatment under Part IV, before proceeding against the patient's wishes.

The A & E nurse should be familiar with the various provisions of the Mental Health Act (1983) as it affects A & E, and should always have a readily available supply of section papers, particularly section 4.

Evaluation

If a mentally disturbed patient has gone through the department with the minimum of fuss and into the appropriate treatment facility, the care given may be evaluated as successful. However, if there has been violence, it is important to look at what happened and why to see if there was a failure of care or whether in the end the patient was just so disturbed that violence was inevitable. If the patient has absconded from A & E, this also needs critical examination in order that the reasons for such a failure may be identified. If it was because there were not enough nurses on duty to keep adequate watch on the patient, then questions have to be asked of nursing management whose responsibility it is to staff the unit. If, however, the person in charge on that shift failed to detail a nurse to stay with the patient, even though sufficient nurses were available, then that person's awareness of what is involved in the care of psychiatric patients is called into question, and perhaps with it the department's attitude to this problem.

Table 17.1
Summary of Mental Health Act (1983)

Legislation	Criteria	Application	Medical Recommendations	Effect
Section 4. Admission for assessment in an emergency.	Admission for assessment required as a matter of urgent necessity.	Nearest relative or Approved Social Worker (ASW) Pt. must be seen by applicant during the 24 hours before application is made.	One written recommendation by any doctor, but if possible, one with previous knowledge of the patient.	Pt. detained for a max. of 72 hours unless 2nd medical opinion given and received by hospital management in that period. Provisions of Part IV on consent to treatment do not apply.
Section 136. Mentally disordered persons in public places.	If a PC finds a person in a public place who appears to be suffering from a mental disorder and is in immediate need of care or control.	A Police Officer	Nil	Person can be taken to place of safety to be interviewed by ASW or doctor, e.g. A & E or Police Station. Maximum 72 hours.
Section 135. Warrant to search for and remove patient.	There is reasonable cause to suspect that a person believed to be	ASW to a JP (on oath)	Nil	PC, ASW and doctor can enter patient's premises and remove him or her to a place of

			unable to care for him or herself and lives alone.
Section 2. Admission for assessment.	Mental disorder warranting detention in hospital for assessment and treatment. The patient ought to be detained in interests of own health and safety or for the protection of others.	Nearest relative and ASW who must interview Pt.	Two doctors, one of whom must be approved under Section 12. Doctors not to be from same hospital.	Patient detained for maximum of 28 days. Part IV applies for treatment without consent.
Section 3. Admission for treatment.	Mental illness or severe impairment, psychopathic disorder or mental impairment of a nature or degree which makes medical treatment in hospital appropriate.	As for Section 2, but ASW cannot make an application if the nearest relative objects.	As for Section 2.	Patient detained for maximum of 6 months, renewable for a further 6, then for 1 year at a time.

Adapted from *A Practical Guide to Mental Health Law*, MIND (1983)

References and Further Reading

Cooper D. (1980). *The Language of Madness*. Harmondsworth: Pelican.
Dubin W. R., Stolberg R. (1981). *Emergency Psychiatry for the House Officer*. Lancaster: MTP Press Ltd.
Gostin L. (1983). *A Practical Guide to Mental Health Law*. London: MIND.
Mitchell R. G. (1983). *Breakdown: Commonsense Psychiatry for Nurses*. London: Nursing Times Publications.
Soreff S. M. (1981). *Management of the Psychiatric Emergency*. New York: John Wiley & Son.

Chapter 18

THE DIFFICULT PROBLEMS THAT NOBODY ELSE WANTS

Most A & E departments have their share of 'regulars', the frequent attenders who are constantly turning up, often because nobody else can think of what to do with them. They include the itinerant travellers, people seeking admission and/or drugs, people with the Munchausen syndrome, vagrant alcoholics and 'dossers', and people suffering from psychopathic personality disorders that do not benefit from psychiatric treatment.

It is worth looking at some of these problem areas in detail, as the difficulties that some of these individuals can cause are out of all proportion to the numbers involved.

NFA ... The Person With Nowhere To Go

The dramatic decline in the amount of privately rented accommodation in cities has greatly exacerbated the problems of homelessness that are encountered by an ever increasing number of people. NFA can be taken as meaning not just people with 'no fixed abode', but also the inhabitants of hostels and cheap lodging houses, people fresh out of prison and people just passing through.

Within this group, alcohol is one major problem that affects all others. The prognosis for the 'Skid Row' alcoholic, drinking the day away in 'schools' with fellow dossers on the waste and parklands of towns and cities, is very poor indeed.

The dossers form a hard core of A & E regulars. Students often ask 'Surely something can be done for these people?' Society answers by locking them in prison for short sentences due to their drunken behaviour in public, which can often be quite aggressive. Most of the agencies involved with dossers, however, admit that this is a waste of time, not benefitting the individuals concerned and merely adding to the overcrowding problems in gaols.

There is no easy answer to the problem of drunken vagrancy. Cook

(1975) after many years working with alcoholic vagrants in London writes: 'One certainly has the feeling . . . that Skid Row has the capacity to absorb any amount of research and social work endeavour, and to remain untouched by it. There is in the Skid Row air as it were a notion of defiance and hopelessness either part of which (or the combination of which) makes reaching out to and helping individuals . . . extremely difficult.'

The use of arguments, such as 'Surely you would be better off if . . .', to try to persuade a vagrant to seek help is considered by Cook to be useless on many occasions due to this air of defiance, this desire to stay outside and fight the system. Nurses' practical experience in A & E unfortunately tends to confirm Cook's pessimistic view.

The A & E nurse will encounter the dosser when he (the majority of dossers are male, although there are homeless women too) is ill as he is very unlikely to have a GP, when he has fallen over drunk causing injuries to himself such as scalp lacerations, or when a member of the public dials 999 for an ambulance for a dosser who has passed out in a public place.

A full assessment should be carried out on reception in A & E, paying particular attention to level of consciousness and airway. Head injury is a common problem, but due to the effects of alcohol extremely difficult to assess. Full level of consciousness and pupil observations should be carried out at regular intervals. It is important to also check for hypothermia, especially in winter.

If there are no immediate interventions needed, the patient is best laid for his own safety on his side on a mattress on the floor, under observation until he has slept off his alcohol sufficiently to leave.

Aggressive behaviour is unfortunately common due to the alcohol and is best dealt with in the usual way (see p. 267), with the police being called to evict the patient if, for example, upon sobering up somewhat, he decides to refuse to leave even though fit. A & E departments are not night shelters for vagrant alcoholics; once a person is fit to go, then they must go.

Although this may seem a hard policy on a cold night in February, the nurse should ask what exactly would be achieved by allowing somebody to stay the night in A & E simply because they said they had nowhere else to go. An alcoholic who has sobered up after a binge in the local park is suffering from far deeper social, psychological and economic problems than a free night in A & E can solve. A more constructive long-term approach is to try to forge links with the local voluntary services working in the field, and with the DHSS and the Social Work department of the hospital so that advice about helpful points of contact with these agencies may be given. There is something of the stick and carrot approach about this, but it is the best long-term solution given the state of the personal social services at present and the multiple problems that are associated with the vagrant alcoholic.

Psychopathic Disorder

'Psychopath' is a term often bandied about in general conversation but usually, like the term schizophrenic, in a totally inappropriate way. Mitchell (1983) quotes McCord's description 'The psychopath is an asocial, aggressive, highly impulsive person, who feels little or no guilt, and is unable to form lasting bonds of friendship with other human beings' and then goes on to add to his definition: they have '. . . an inability to learn from past experience or punishment and a superficial, often sexual, attractiveness'.

Such individuals often live turbulent and troubled lives, satisfying their needs by a whole range of strategies varying from obtaining their objectives by simply hitting somebody over the head and taking whatever they want, to manipulating an individual (or the system) for their own ends. Their mood can change from one of apparent contrition and regret to extreme aggression and violence in an instant, the constant factor being a desire to get their own way regardless of anybody else and what is right or wrong.

What sort of problems do psychopathic individuals cause in A & E? The more manipulative and passive psychopaths often take drug overdoses and practice DSH. Often they attend A & E in an apparently distressed state claiming that if they are not admitted to a psychiatric ward immediately they will commit suicide. Attention-seeking behaviour is indulged in freely, such as taking their overdose or cutting themselves in front of a queue of people.

The more aggressive psychopath turns up in A & E often with injuries associated with a fight and frequently under the influence of alcohol or else demanding drugs. Their potential for violence is high, especially when they realise that they are not going to get what they want. Disruptive behaviour is common and mental illness is frequently claimed.

In dealing with such a disturbed individual, the first step is to recognise that they are not suffering from a psychotic state which has deprived them of insight. They are fully aware of what they are doing and consequently are fully responsible for the consequences of their actions in A & E. Disruptive behaviour should be dealt with firmly and promptly by asking the person to desist. If they refuse, the danger is that by making too much fuss, the nurse will be merely rewarding the behaviour and thereby leading to its likely repetition. The aim is to deny them the attention that they crave, even if they are swallowing Valium tablets two at a time in front of the queue. They know exactly what they are doing and must take the consequences (usually little more than a long sleep) and attempts to physically restrain them would only lead to staff getting hurt.

Limits have to be set for such individuals for the protection of other patients in the department whose treatment may be adversely affected by disruptive acting out behaviour. The limits of acceptable behaviour should be clearly stated at the beginning of the attendance (e.g. no shouting, running around the department or intruding into certain areas) and if the person goes beyond those limits, they should be removed from A & E by the police. Female nurses are just as likely as male nurses to be punched or kicked by aggressive psychopaths.

Munchausen's Syndrome

This syndrome was first recognised in 1951 by Asher and according to Enoch and Trethowan (1979) consists of individuals 'who obtain admission to hospital with apparently acute illness supported by a plausible but dramatic history which is later found to be full of falsifications. They are subsequently discovered to have attended and deceived staff at many other hospitals and frequently to have discharged themselves against medical advice, often following arguments while under investigation or following a surgical operation.'

Such is the highly mobile nature of these individuals that it is almost always to A & E that they present and, unless picked up early, can consume great amounts of time and energy (and money) having their 'illnesses' treated.

There are five principal types of Munchausen's syndrome:

1. *The Acute Abdominal Type.* They will manifest acute abdominal symptoms, and some may swallow objects such as razor blades and safety pins in order to obtain the surgery and hospitalisation they crave. In well-documented cases individuals have obtained well over 100 admissions and laparotomies numbered in double figures.

2. *The Haemorrhagic Type.* This is characterised by complaints of bleed-

ing from various orifices: haematurea (coupled with renal colic in order to obtain pethidine), haemoptysis and haematemesis are common. Self-inflicted wounds with needles or razor blades are commonly used to provide the blood to make the samples realistic, e.g. a finger is nicked so that drops of blood can be squeezed into a urine specimen or the back of the tongue may be cut to lend colouring to haemoptysis.

3. *The Neurological Type.* This type of the syndrome is characterised by very convincing (and some not so convincing) epileptic fits or complaints of migraine.

4. *The Cardiac Type.* This type is characterised by a very convincing display of central chest pain that shows considerable knowledge of medical textbooks. Many such patients know that IV diamorphine is administered for chest pain, hence their behaviour.

5. *The Psychiatric Type.* Imitating various forms of mental illness in order to gain admission to psychiatric hospitals is another manifestation of the syndrome.

Some patients maintain a consistent story; others will change their symptoms as they travel. In trying to understand these people, we should not expect a single simple answer. In some cases obtaining drugs is undoubtedly a major feature (e.g. the chest pain type and those feigning renal colic), but there is much more to it than this. They are often attention-seeking, very immature and psychopathic in personality. For others admission to hospital is a way of escaping from the demands of having to cope with the real world outside.

In many Munchausen's patients there appears to be a strong streak of masochism. This fits well into the abdominal type of the syndrome, as they undergo repeated self-induced wounding and may also practice self-mutilation. It has been found that tolerance to unpleasant diagnostic procedures may be high, and their pain thresholds are also high. It is difficult to explain their desire for mutilation, be it by the hand of the surgeon or (sometimes) their own hand, without including a masochistic element in their personality.

The following list of observations should alert the nurse to the possibility that the patient is suffering from Munchausen's syndrome.

1. Any patient presenting alone, who is non-resident in the catchment area of the hospital, who has no apparent injury.
2. A vague reason for being in the area that cannot be readily substantiated, e.g. a long distance lorry driver says he has left his lorry at a lorry park.

3. If a discreet search of their clothing and effects reveals inconsistencies in their story such as a different name or address from that given, or evidence of having come from a different part of the country from that which they have stated. There may be evidence of their last port of call such as hospital name tags inside clothes and pyjamas, or evidence of being on the road such as shaving equipment or a change of underwear in a jacket pocket.

4. If the person is known to the A & E department in their previous locality. Check that there is such an address or GP as that given in the area.

5. If there are signs of recent IV sites or cut downs. Multiple abdominal scars should rate a very high probability of Munchausen's, if points 1 and 2 are found to be present.

6. If the patient's description of their symptoms is just a little too perfect or textbookish. In practice very few people ever have all the symptoms in the textbook for any given illness.

7. If the patient's manner and behaviour, especially when they think they are not being observed, gives cause for suspicion.

8. If the patient asks for analgesia by the name of a drug.

9. If there is a circular about the person in your 'black book'.

What is the course of action when little or no physical signs of illness can be found, and the staff are reasonably sure of the diagnosis of Munchausen's syndrome? The basic health problem here is undoubtedly a mental one, however, experience has shown that when offered psychiatric help (except in the case of the psychiatric type), the patient will often abscond and move on to try elsewhere.

There are differing opinions about whether to confront the person in A & E with their diagnosis. It is the author's belief that they should be confronted and informed that all hospitals in the area will be circulated at once with their descriptions and details. This should be done over the telephone immediately for your local A & E departments. The rationale that lies behind this policy is that while they are resistant to most forms of psychiatric help that have been tried, the best chance is to deny them the attention that they seek by ensuring that they are discovered as soon as possible in other areas, thereby removing the rewards that the individual gets from their abnormal behaviour. Experimental evidence suggests that this is the most effective way of suppressing unwanted behaviour as has been referred to before in this book (see p. 22). In addition it will also save the hard-pressed NHS considerable time and money. Enoch and Trethowan come to similar conclusions in their detailed review of the problem, hoping for a decline in the behaviour by denying the rewards that are associated with it.

Such a policy requires cooperation between departments on a national scale to exchange information on these sad individuals. Computer technology could lead to the development of a central registry with each A & E department having access via a terminal. The scale of the problem, given the itinerant nature of these people, is national; therefore the solution should reflect this characteristic of the problem. Meanwhile departments are recommended to insure maximum distribution of information concerning Munchausen's patients they come across.

Violence and Aggression

The origins of aggression and violence in the human species are the subject of much debate. One group of theories suggests that aggression comes from within, that it is an integral part of the human condition. Freud postulated that there was a basic aggression drive within all humans that was an instinct. This view was however rejected by later theorists in the Freudian tradition who developed a frustration–aggression hypothesis based on the idea that preventing a person from obtaining a goal leads to frustration and the focussing of aggression on to the blocking object.

An alternative view of aggression sees it as a learned response no different from any other, so that together with violent actions, it is learned by observation and imitation. The more they are rewarded, the more they will be reinforced and consequently the more likely they are to recur. Bandura's classic experiments (1979) showed how children learned to be violent and the reader is referred to Schachter's work (see p. 16) for a discussion of the emotional behaviour that is involved in aggression.

Violence occurs in many different settings and with many different types of actors. The following list enumerates just some of them.

1. Domestic/family violence.
2. Associated with organic disease, e.g. post-head injury or hypoglycaemic state.
3. Associated with psychosis, e.g. schizophrenia.
4. Due to the effects of drugs, e.g. hallucinogenics and alcohol.
5. Professional violence, the mugger or the soldier.
6. Groups such as football hooligans.

7. Sexual violence, rape.
8. Individual loss of control—violence in response to a situation, heavily influenced by role playing and stereotypes.

The victims of all these types of aggression and violence, and their perpetrators, end up in A & E. An understanding of the psychological processes that are involved in aggressive and violent behaviour will help us to help our patients, and prevent us from being counted among the next victims ourselves.

It is very rare for violence to erupt spontaneously without any warning and reason. There are opportunities, therefore, for intervention before violence occurs which will allow nurses to defuse the situation and lower the temperature.

A major cause of aggression in A & E, compounding any of the situations listed above, is a patient's unrealistic expectations. The classic one that most A & E nurses will be familiar with is the length of the queue to see the doctor. Patients often expect instant attention and are not prepared to wait for more serious cases to be seen. A simple device that is very effective is a blackboard kept at the reception desk informing patients, as they book in, of how long approximately they will have to wait. This dispels unrealistic expectations at once, and allows people to make arrangements, if they have to, for a long stay. If there is going to be an argument about the waiting times, it is better that it occur at the beginning of a visit to A & E rather than after somebody has spent 2 hours or so in the queue building up their frustration and anger.

Departments should think about the provision of facilities to keep people amused while they are waiting; toys, magazines, piped radio, a TV or a video (well secured to the wall!), a public phone and a drinks machine would all be desirable. Generally nurses should look at the waiting environment provided in A & E and ask if it is really satisfactory—especially if patients have to wait there for 3 or 4 hours with a painful injury.

If, however, you are confronted by an aggressive individual, what then? There are several things that you can do to prevent the situation from getting out of hand. First, keep your voice to its normal pitch and volume. When shouted at, it is easy to shout back, but don't. It only raises the temperature immediately. There is nothing wrong with telling yourself repeatedly to control yourself; it is a feedback mechanism that works.

Body positioning is critically important. Stand just a little more than an arm's length (the patient's arm) away. This is far enough to give you the chance to escape any sudden grab or punch, but not so far away as to suggest disinterest in the patient's problem. Standing too close, on the other hand, crowds the person's individual space and is very threatening, so try to keep this arm's length distance between you and the patient at all times.

Your posture should be slightly oblique to the patient. Standing square on is very confrontational, especially if you have your arms in the traditional nursing position of folded across the chest.

The correct stance, according to Moran (1984), is with one leg slightly behind the other. The back leg should be the dominant one and should be straight with your weight fully on it, while the leading leg should be slightly flexed at the knee. This position poses minimal threat, but coupled with the distance you have placed between yourself and the aggressor, gives you the best chance of avoiding a kick or a blow.

Moran points out that in this particular situation, eye to eye contact can be construed as very provocative and should therefore be avoided. He recommends that the nurse should concentrate their attention at a point about level with the second shirt button down. This still conveys interest and gives you the best chance of seeing a punch or grab with your peripheral vision while not threatening the aggressor with direct eyeball to eyeball contact. (See Figs. 18.1, 18.2 and 18.3.)

Finally you should be aware of any suspicious bulges in jacket pockets that may be potential weapons such as bottles, and of any potential weapons in the immediate environment of the patient. Do not carry pointed scissors and, whatever sort you do use, keep them well out of view. They have been used on a number of occasions to assault nursing staff. The practice of wearing a stethoscope draped around the back of the neck should be frowned upon for the same reason.

Verbal contact with the patient will often allow the situation to be brought under control. Try to avoid an immediate confrontational attitude—a them and us situation. Explain that you are there to try to help. What can you do? What is the patient's problem?

The person should be interviewed individually if possible, without friends and relatives who are often the cause of more trouble than the patient. When a group of rowdy individuals brings one of their mates to A & E, the best policy is to ask the rest to leave. They will accomplish nothing in the department except be disruptive and endeavour to impress each other with acts of bravado, depending on the pecking order in the group. Such behaviour is well documented in studies of group violence. Allowing such a group to remain in the department will only lead to trouble, therefore they should be asked to leave

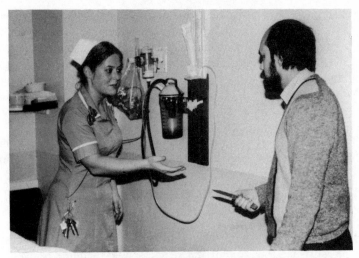

Fig. 18.1   The patient in A & E with a weapon. The wrong
approach: the nurse has allowed the patient to get between her
and the outside of the cubicle. She is holding out her hand
demanding the knife and she is making eye to eye contact. This is
confronting and threatening to the patient and may cause him to
respond violently and he may use the knife to inflict serious harm.

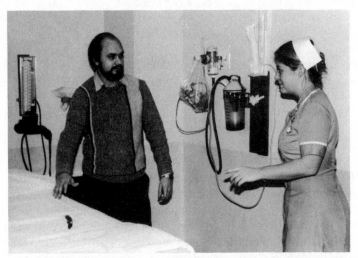

Fig. 18.2   The right approach. The nurse is keeping to the outside
of the cubicle and is asking the patient to place the weapon on
neutral territory before attempting to remove it. She is keeping at
a safe distance (arm's length) and avoiding eye to eye contact.

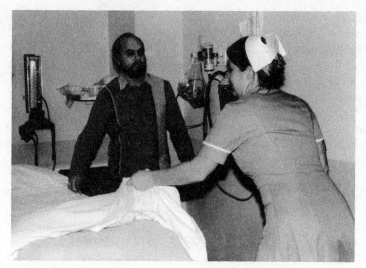

Fig. 18.3 If attacked with a weapon, the nurse should try to smother it with a blanket or anything else available, while retreating rapidly to safety and calling for help.

and if they refuse, the matter referred to the security service or the police.

One of the most effective ways of defusing a situation is simply by passing on information. People are far less likely to get angry if they know what is going on, how long they will have to wait, and why.

However, there are some situations in which, despite all these measures, violence still erupts or, to be more precise, passes from being verbal to physical. In many cases, the patient will smash some physical objects, throw a chair at a wall or window, but then become calmer again having 'let off steam' as it were. Therefore, if a patient indulges in an outburst against property, they are best left to break whatever it is they have in mind (within reason) as probably that will be the end of the episode and if you do intervene the result will be a violent struggle in which you will become the object of the person's aggression. Broken windows are easier to repair than broken staff nurses' arms.

The police should, however, be contacted and asked for assistance, for the staff may yet become the objects of the person's violence. Furthermore, prosecution for serious damage to hospital property should be the policy of the department.

If the person challenges a male member of staff to a fight, going perhaps through the ritual of removing the coat, issuing threats and insults, then violence is less likely to occur, providing the situation is handled correctly. Allow the person to have a 'moral' victory by backing off. The ritual having been fulfilled (Mungham 1977, Marsh 1975), physical contact is unlikely. While the patient is boasting of his victory and swaggering around the department, the police can be on the way. Remember it's usually the winner of the last battle that wins the war.

At the end of the day, however, a direct assault on a member of staff may occur. When intervention is needed (as in such a situation), the basic premises of military strategy still hold good, i.e. concentration of force in time and space coupled with the element of surprise. This means that you should insure sufficient pairs of hands to do the job (ideally at least 4 people), plan the move to be simultaneous so as to overwhelm the person, and if possible detract his attention or come from the rear. This way the risk of injury to staff and patient is minimised. Although the situation in which direct physical intervention is required is unpredictable and, therefore, hard and fast rules cannot be made, the nurse would do well to adhere to these basic principles.

A final comment on aggression and violence in A & E—all incidents should be documented, and there should be in-service training for all A & E nursing staff in the skills required to handle aggressive patients.

References and Further Reading

Enoch M. D., Trethowan W. H. (1979). *Uncommon Psychiatric Syndromes*. Bristol: John Wright and Sons.

Bandura K. (1979). In *Introduction to Psychology* (Hilgard E., Atkinson R., Atkinson R. C., eds.), pp. 322–3. New York: Harcourt, Brace Jovanovitch.

Cook T. (1975). *Vagrant Alcoholics*. London: Routledge & Kegan Paul.

Marsh P. (1975). Understanding Aggro. *New Society*, 3.4.75.

Mitchell R. G. (1983). *Breakdown: Commonsense Psychiatry for Nurses*. London: Nursing Times Publications.

Moran J. (1984). Response and Responsibility, *Nursing Times*, 80 (14): 28–31.

Mungham G. (1977). The Sociology of Violence, *New Society*, 13.10.77.

Chapter 19

SEXUAL PROBLEMS IN A & E

Sexually Transmitted Disease

Patients sometimes present at A & E, often in a very distressed condition, thinking that they are suffering from some form of sexually transmitted disease. It is essential to know something of the more common types and their presenting symptoms in order that an assessment of the patient's problems may be made.

Figure 19.1 illustrates the proportional split of the different types of disease that were reported in the UK in 1982. It can be seen that non-specific genital infections are the most common (142 066 cases) followed by gonorrhoea (58 762 cases). These two diseases are rapidly increasing in incidence, but the biggest rate of increase of all is genital herpes (14 836 cases) although levels of genital herpes in the UK are considerably lower than in the USA where it is talked of as an epidemic in some quarters.

Patients usually come to A & E when the local department of genito-urinary medicine is closed, and very often refuse to give details of their complaint to the receptionist, either out of embarrassment or because they cannot find the words to express their problem, without resorting to vulgar terms which they are often unwilling to use in front of the receptionist.

The department should have a policy to the effect that if a patient does not wish to disclose the nature of their complaint, rather than have a receptionist pursue the matter to their embarrassment, a member of the nursing staff (preferably of the same sex) should be asked to talk to the patient.

In assessing the patient, privacy is important, and the nurse should try to set the patient at their ease and then ask them to explain the nature of their problem. Many people are not familiar with the medical words used to describe sexual function and anatomy, therefore the language used may involve slang and some rather crude terms. It is important to obtain a description of the symptoms—how long they have been present for and how they relate to the patient's sexual behaviour over the last 4

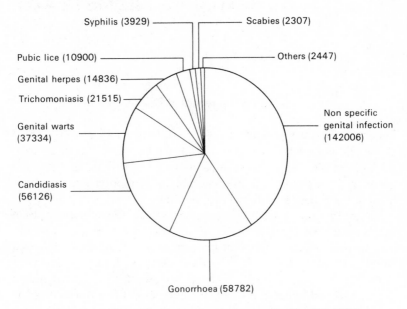

Fig. 19.1   *Sexually transmitted diseases in the UK, 1982.*

weeks. If the patient has been monogamous during that period, the clear implication is that their partner has not, which can have a very damaging effect on their relationship. As in other illnesses, the psychological and social sides of the problem must not be overlooked, and great care and sensitivity is required in talking, for instance, to a married woman who has suddenly developed a vaginal discharge, two weeks after her lorry driver husband has returned from a trip to Europe.

The two most common complaints that will be heard are a discharge (vaginal or urethral) or ulceration of the genitalia. The significance of these complaints is as follows:

1. *Urethral discharge in males.* This is almost always pathological and can be broadly classified into either gonococcal or non-gonococcal, the most common non-gonococcal causes being *Chlamydia trachomatis*, *Trichomonas vaginalis* and *Candida albicans* organisms. If uncircumcised males are suffering from Candida infection, they will reveal the site of the

infection clearly upon retraction of the foreskin. However the origin of the discharge in the other conditions is not so easily located.

A useful test is to ask the man to pass 60–120 ml of urine into a glass container, and then to finish off passing his urine into another glass container. If there is infection of the anterior urethra, the first specimen will be hazy, containing threads or specks of pus, while the second specimen will be clear. If, however, they are both hazy this indicates that the infection involves other parts of the urinary tract, e.g. cystitis or nephritis.

2. *Vaginal discharge.* This can be either pathological or non-pathological. Some degree of discharge from the vagina occurs in all women, the amount varying along a continuum. It is important to ascertain, therefore, what the normal discharge is like and why this condition is different. The women should be reminded that a normal vaginal discharge may increase and be only noticed premenstrually, at time of ovulation or when using the contraceptive pill or an IUD. A discharge therefore does not automatically imply a disease process.

If the discharge is pathological in origin, the most likely cause is *Candida albicans* (which some authorities do not consider to be an exclusively sexually transmitted disease), while other organisms that might be responsible are *Neisseria gonorrhoeae, Trichomonas vaginalis* and *Chlamydia trachomatis.* Cervical lesions may also produce a vaginal discharge whether they are infective (herpes or warts) or not (neoplasm, polyps).

3. *Genital ulceration.* In practice, there tend to be two types of ulcer found, ulcers that are multiple and painful (usually herpes) and those that occur singly and are painless (usually syphilis).

Diagnosis of the infecting organism on clinical findings is very uncertain, therefore careful microbiological examination and culture are required, which is why departments of genito-urinary medicine usually insist that A & E departments do not treat these cases, but rather refer them on to their clinic. It is a famous dictum that there is no such thing as an emergency in venereology, and while there may be a lot of truth in this from the physical point of view, it may not be so true from the psychological angle.

Standard policy is to not treat the patient but to tell them instead to attend the clinic the following day or the next Monday, and it is probably true to say that no physical harm will come to the patient. However, when nurses are passing this information on or reinforcing what the Casualty Officer has said, they need to remember that the patient will be very anxious and considerable reassurance is needed that this wait is for the best. Abstinence from sexual activity is to be strongly recommended until attending clinic when it is next open.

One of the most important reasons for the patient attending the clinic rather than receiving treatment in A & E is the need for the patient's sexual partners to be traced—a role that A & E units cannot take on. Various forms of sexually transmitted disease produce no symptoms, or symptoms which can be and are ignored. For example, rectal gonorrhoea is often symptomless and, given the often multiple nature of homosexual encounters, it is therefore very important indeed to trace contacts as they may not know that they have been infected. (If symptoms do appear they consist of anal pain and discomfort, painful defaecation and a blood-stained or purulent discharge.) Oropharyngeal gonorrhoea likewise is often asymptomatic.

The reader will be aware that there are various forms of sexually transmitted disease besides those described so far (e.g. genital warts, 37 000 cases per year), but this is not a textbook on venereology. What matters is that the nurse can show sympathy and understanding for what is a very distressing condition *for the patient*, and that the nurse is able to assess that the most likely cause of the problem is sexual transmission, and therefore that the most appropriate place of treatment is not A & E but the out-patient clinic of the department of genito-urinary medicine. Telephone calls in the middle of the night are another manifestation of the anxiety felt by persons who think they may have acquired such a disease. Such calls should be dealt with tactfully and with due understanding, the patient being advised to attend the appropriate clinic and abstain from sexual activity meanwhile.

Homosexuality

It is important for the A & E nurse to define their attitude towards homosexuality which, in fact, is not a sexual 'problem' but rather a sexual choice. (It is discussed here for lack of a more appropriate section.) A significant proportion of the population is homosexual or bisexual, and as a consequence a significant proportion of A & E patients will be 'gay'. In many cases this probably will not be recognised, but in other situations the person may display behaviour that is more in keeping with their sexual orientation, in a way that is perfectly natural to them. This is a sexual orientation that the nurse has no right to censure.

Society still broadly disapproves of homosexuality, which places many homosexuals under great pressure. Some are more able to live with these pressures than others, while others again are just unable to come to terms at all with their homosexual tendencies, especially if they are married. The result is a great deal of stress in the lives of many homosexuals which, coupled with the often transient nature of homosexual relationships and, therefore, a lack of stability and support, may lead to a higher incidence of unhappiness and anxiety than in other sections of the population. Homosexuals, for instance, appear to have a higher than normal incidence of DSH. Such a hypothesis is untested and probably untestable, but it should act as food for thought for the A & E nurse.

The nurse must lend an understanding and sympathetic ear if required by a gay patient. We are not in A & E to make moral judgements about patients' sexual orientations, or to judge them by heterosexual standards. Our job is to help people (to help themselves, according to Orem) not to pass judgement on them.

As a postscript to this brief discussion, much has been said about the incidence of AIDS (Acquired Immunity Deficiency Syndrome) among homosexuals in the USA. By March 1984, 3600 cases had been notified in the USA and 108 by December 1984 in the UK (RCN, 1985). Of the US cases 71·3% were among homosexuals, the next most common group being IV drug abusers with 17·4%. Mortality over a two year period approaches 100%. Anxious midnight telephone calls to A & E should be dealt with sympathetically with these figures in mind. The number of the local Gay Switchboard should be available to pass on to callers in the small hours or, of course, the Samaritans, if they are very distressed. The risk of AIDS transmission via blood should reinforce the need for nursing staff to observe the strictest precautions in disposing of sharps. Guidelines on caring for patients with AIDS are available from the RCN.

Genital Trauma

The sexual acts that people perform in the privacy of their own homes are their own business. However, some practices can occasionally have unfortunate consequences which lead the person, with great reluctance and embarrassment, to the local A & E department.

A common problem is that of a foreign body that has either been retained in the rectum, vagina or urethra, or damage done to any of these organs by such a foreign body.

In dealing with a rectal foreign body, the patient may admit to what is causing the problem (e.g. a carrot or a sex-aid such as a vibrator) or to what was responsible for the injuries sustained (e.g. a glass or bottle that has broken leading to lacerations of the rectum and anal area) which makes treatment much easier. However, such is the embarrassment felt that the patient may not bring themselves to admit the truth. It is essential to bear this in mind when somewhat reluctant individuals walk into A & E complaining they have not been able to open their bowels for several days or that they are bleeding rectally, or simply complaining of abdominal pain. In such cases, rupture of the bowel is possible with disastrous consequences. Laparotomy to remove the offending object may be necessary; vibrators have been known to reach the transverse colon. Severe rectal damage may be caused by practices that involve inserting the forearm into the rectum; smooth muscle relaxant drugs are abused in conjunction with this practice, e.g. glycerin trinitrate.

A wide variety of foreign bodies may be removed from the vagina, with or without the woman's admission of their presence.

Urethral trauma can occur from the passing of objects such as straws or the flexible inside part of a biro. Fresh bleeding from the urethra should raise this possibility even though the patient may not admit to such a practice.

Trauma to the external genitals may be the result of sadomasochistic practices, or may be accidental. An unlikely story together with the patient's unease should make the former cause more likely in the nurse's mind, but nurses should treat the injuries at their face value, and not be too concerned with how they were caused (unless there is a possibility that they were inflicted against the person's will, in which case discreet probing when alone with the patient should be undertaken).

A common injury is the zip injury to the penis which can be exquisitely painful. Generous analgesia with Entonox will greatly facilitate freeing the penis from the zip. If swelling is present, ice packs should be applied and lignocaine gel may be of help. Uncircumcised males who have a tight foreskin run the risk during their first sexual encounters of the foreskin becoming so retracted that it will not resume its normal anatomical position, acting as a tight constriction around the end of the penis leading to swelling and oedema (paraphimosis). This is a very alarming condition and, as with all such sexual problems, the nurse should display great tact and reassurance in dealing with the patient. Ice packs to reduce the swelling together with the use of lignocaine gel will in most cases allow the foreskin to be manipulated back to its normal position. The patient should be advised about circumcision.

Relatively minor lacerations to the penis can bleed profusely, and the patient may well limp into A & E after several hours of bleeding. Even after suturing, bleeding may occur. Ice packs and firm manual pressure are recommended, although it may take some time to finally stop the bleeding from what is a very vascular organ.

Bruising and swelling of the scrotum are often seen after accidents and are best treated with ice and a scrotal support. The nurse should be alerted, however, by the young man who says that he has severe pain but has no apparent injury as this is the classical presentation of torsion testis which, if not promptly relieved by surgery, can lead to a gangrenous testicle due to the impairment of the blood supply. This should be treated with a high priority to see the Casualty Officer.

One final problem that may occur, although not usually associated with genital trauma (although it may be), is the patient who refuses to undress for no apparent reason. The nurse may be dealing with a case of transexuality or transvestism. Transexuality involves a person who wishes to live like a member of the opposite sex because they consider that that is their appropriate sex. Transvestism is more in the nature of a fetish for women's clothes. In the former case, the person underneath the clothes may be of the opposite gender to the outer clothes, while in the latter case very often the outer clothes conform, but underneath a jacket and trousers may be concealed a petticoat, suspender belt or other female clothing. The patient's extreme anxiety may be understood in such a situation and the nurse should ensure that as few people as possible know about the patient's predicament. This will build up the trust and cooperation that is needed to treat the injuries sustained by the patient most effectively.

Occasionally cases of genital mutilation may be seen in persons craving to be of the opposite sex, which in the author's own experience have ranged from a pair of tights tied tightly around the base of the penis and scrotum (in the hope that 'Like a wart tied with string, it would all drop off'—the result was only an agonisingly painful blue scrotum) to an attempt to shoot off, with a shotgun, the relevant piece of anatomy.

In dealing with the sort of problems described above, the nurse may have feelings ranging from surprise to complete revulsion. But a non-judgemental attitude is the key to helping the patient, which means that feelings and emotions must be kept under control and not communicated to the patient who, as can be imagined, is already in a hypersensitive condition. The sexual aspect of a patient's life is largely ignored in nurse training—perhaps another Victorian legacy of the Nightingale tradition—but in A & E this cannot be, as many of the problems that patients present with are directly sexual in origin, or can be traced at least partly to the stresses and anxieties that have been generated by sexual problems.

References and Further Reading

Adler M. (1984). *The ABC of Sexually Transmitted Diseases*. London: BMJ
RCN (1985). *Nursing Standard* lead article. January 10. London: Royal College of Nursing.

Organisation in A & E

Chapter 20

TEACHING IN A & E

In view of the specialised nature of A & E nursing, there is a great requirement for teaching within the department. Two principle areas may be identified: the basic needs of learners having their first experience of A & E, and the needs of qualified staff to both broaden and deepen their existing knowledge in the ever-changing area of A & E.

Education cannot take place effectively without a planned curriculum, which in its turn requires a clear idea of just what the role and function of the nurse in A & E is. A department must therefore ask itself such basic questions as—what do we see our nurses doing? What are their responsibilities and roles? Where do the limits of their responsibility lie? What conceptual model of nursing are we to use? How do we plan to carry out the process of nursing?

Only when answers to these questions are found can nurses begin to map out the areas that basic learners need to cover, and at the same time, begin to consider appropriate areas to explore with trained staff.

Having laid out the boundaries of the general areas that we wish to cover, the department has effectively laid out its *aims*. The next step is to define specific objectives within those aims, related to the levels at which basic students and qualified staff are expected to function.

For example, plaster of Paris will probably have been mapped out as an area to cover; this has therefore become an aim. The next step is then to define specific objectives which can be measured (or else how will we know if they have been achieved?) concerning the use of POP and relevant to the differing levels of function of basic students and qualified staff.

Objectives for students should then be to have seen how POP is applied and to know why it is applied for different injuries to various parts of the body. The students should be able to list these. Furthermore, if Orem's model of nursing is being used, we would also expect the student to be aware of the self-care problems that the patient will have at home and of how the nurses can help the patient to overcome these difficulties or self-care deficits.

On the level of newly recruited trained staff to the department, we may set objectives such as understanding the theory of POP application, having sufficient supervised practice to be able to apply POPs for certain listed injuries, and being able to explore potential self-care deficits with patients before discharge in order to give the appropriate advice and make whatever arrangements are needed to allow the patient to make good the self-care deficit.

At the stage of setting aims and objectives, it is essential that there be close liaison with the School of Nursing. Otherwise the situation may arise where the department staff feel that the school is teaching irrelevant information, while the school staff teach procedures in ways that are not carried out in the department. How often does a frustrated student get told 'I don't care what they taught you in the school, this is how we do it here'? Such contradictory instruction is inevitably demoralising for the student as it breeds a feeling of 'No matter what I do it's always wrong'.

In view of the specialised nature of A & E, the school of nursing should have a tutor solely responsible for the A & E part of basic nurse education who has substantial A & E experience. Only with such experience will the school's educational effort be relevant to the needs of basic learners and at the same time have sufficient 'street credibility' among the A & E staff as to be acceptable. A nurse tutor with no background in A & E will encounter difficulties with A & E staff if the tutor tries to tell the staff what should be taught in A & E. No matter how good their ideas may be, their lack of acceptance by the A & E staff, due to their lack of experience, will prove a fatal handicap.

While there is a need, therefore, for a tutor in the school with credibility in the department, there is also a need for the department to have educational credibility in the school. Credibility is a two-edged sword. There should be close liaison and joint planning of aims and objectives together with a departmental input into the formal teaching programme of the school. The nomination of a member of the A & E staff to be responsible for school liaison is an idea that should be considered.

With the modular system of teaching now in use, there is usually a period of several days formal school-based instruction before students come to A & E. Departmental involvement is a good idea at this stage in order to familiarise the students with the department and ensure realistic expectations.

Within the A & E experience, formal teaching is not always feasible, especially when the unpredictable nature of the workload is considered. In group teaching, therefore, the need is for flexibility, while in individual teaching great use should be made of the time-honoured principle of 'sitting next to Nelly'.

The sitting next to Nelly principle means learning how to do something by watching somebody else. Many nurses say they cannot teach, but they are in fact teaching every hour of every shift by simply doing their job. Learners will copy them, bad habits and all. Much can be taught to learners by simply getting them to watch what we are doing.

However this in itself is not sufficient, for we must also explain the reasons and principles behind our actions in order that the student may understand the action or nursing intervention sufficiently to adapt it to a differing set of circumstances; very few patients are ever the same. Furthermore, we need to evaluate the effectiveness of our teaching, for as has been said elsewhere—it is not what is taught that counts but what is learnt. The student should be able to explain the whys and wherefores of a nursing intervention and demonstrate it to the satisfaction of the qualified member of staff before it can be said that learning has occurred.

Teaching by the sitting next to Nelly principle is the responsibility of all the staff in the department, and one hopes not to see students standing around while trained staff are actually performing various interventions. Those students should be watching!

Teaching in group situations is economical in terms of time—you only have to explain something once to six students in a group rather than six times to them individually—and it also permits group discussion which is an opportunity for bringing up new ideas and exploring how students feel about various matters. It does, however, require certain skills to lead a group teaching session.

The length of time available for a group session is very variable, therefore the nurse must be able to break down A & E theory into chunks of varying length so as to make maximum use of the times that are available.

This is not the situation for a formal lecture, but rather for an informal discussion with the 'teacher' acting as a discussion leader. There is a need before the start to have certain key points that you want the group to understand at the end, even if they have learnt nothing else, and to make these points the pegs on which you are going to hang the rest of the content of the session.

It is a good idea to pick something fresh in their memories to discuss, such as a patient they have just seen in the department, and then broaden out the discussion to bring in the various aspects of the condition, using the patient as an example to illustrate your points. This use of a real patient as an example will considerably assist learning.

A teacher who is doing all the talking with little feedback from the group is unlikely to be doing much teaching. It is essential to involve the group, question them, and ask them to give examples and to describe things. A judicious mixture of facts thrown in by the teacher and questions fired at specific students, whose answers can be built on and expanded by the teacher or other group members, with perhaps a general discussion at the end, will convey much more information to students than a straight one-way lecture. Never throw out open questions, as you end up with the same one or two people answering them while the rest switch off.

One final need in the department is for learning materials such as books, journals, and a folder with photocopies of relevant articles. Such a resource is of great value in that it permits students to engage in private study when trained staff might be busy elsewhere. Such study can also be coordinated by giving individual members particular aspects of the same problem to explore, so that the whole can be discussed as a group later.

In deciding the areas to be covered by students in A & E, the social and psychological backgrounds to conditions must be included in order that the student may see the person and their problem in their true context, rather than as a piece of malfunctioning anatomy and physiology or simply as another procedure to carry out. The failings of general nurse training in this regard should not be imported into A & E.

With respect to qualified staff, it is clear that there are various procedures not learnt by students that need to be learnt now, such as applying POPs, performing ECGs and suturing. Simply watching other members of staff perform these interventions, the basic sitting next to Nelly method, is not good enough. As in the case of students, there must be proper instruction in the theory of what is involved, supervised practice and finally an assessment of competence. The person responsible for assessment should be a nurse for only nurses are competent to assess nursing competence. The liaison nurse with the school or the specialist A & E tutor are likely people to take on this role of teaching advanced skills and assessing competence.

It is important for the professional development and interest of qualified staff that, in addition to acquiring the skills of A & E nursing practice, they should attend study days and conferences relevant to their field in order to keep up with new ideas and research findings. Is not nursing after all a research-based profession?

A well-informed nursing management will support nurses' attempts to attend conferences by granting study leave or financial assistance, in the belief that such activities give future patients the chance to benefit from improved standards of care and are enhancing the development of nursing as a profession.

In this connection, A & E nurses would be well advised to join the RCN A & E Nursing Forum which produces its own newsletter and organises conferences and study days on a wide variety of A & E-related subjects around the UK.

It would be inappropriate to conclude a chapter on teaching in A & E without mentioning that as nurses we should be teaching our patients all the time. Reference has been made extensively throughout the book to this aspect of nursing intervention, and the A & E nurse should bear this in mind at all times.

Chapter 21

MAJOR DISASTER PLANNING AND RADIATION CASUALTIES

Major Disaster Planning

Major A & E departments are required to have a plan that they can implement in the case of a major disaster, and all A & E nurses should be familiar with their department's plan.

Major disaster plans should not, however, be engraved in tablets of stone, unchangeable and immutable for time eternal. They, like any other human endeavour, can always be improved, especially in the light of experience gained by others in coping with a real incident. A & E departments should, therefore, keep their plans under constant review.

The basic principle that should run through a good plan is that people perform best, especially under stressful conditions, when they are doing the things with which they are most familiar. Thus plans should avoid major changes in work practices and departmental layout, aiming to have the department functioning like an ordinary, although very busy, day as far as possible.

A second key principle is that of flexibility and simplicity. A rigid plan that will cope with all eventualities is not possible as it is not possible to foresee all such eventualities. After all, if disasters could be predicted they could be largely avoided. Simplicity has the virtue of allowing flexibility and also of making for greater staff retention and compliance with content. The more there is in a plan that can go wrong, the more will go wrong.

Within the department, the person who should be in charge is the senior Sister/Charge Nurse on duty, in other words, the person who would normally be in charge. The place for senior nursing management is doing what they normally do—organising the rest of the hospital, providing extra staff where needed and supplying the A & E unit with back-up facilities such as extra equipment, trolleys and pairs of hands.

Once the alert has been received, there is a need to evacuate A & E immediately of all patients, either by sending them to wards or moving them to a holding area (e.g. out-patients clinic), in order to free staff and facilities for casualty reception. A designated disaster ward that will receive all admitted casualties is a good idea, not only for immediate logistic reasons, but also for long-term psychological reasons in the days and weeks after the disaster when its victims have to come to terms with life after serious injury, e.g. loss of a limb.

Many of the patients that attend will be very distressed and tearful, but may be suffering little serious injury. For example, of the 76 hospitalised casualties of the 1983 Harrods bombing, only 14 were admitted. In bombings patients will complain of headaches and deafness. Perforated eardrums may be common due to the blast effect.

Provision should be made for relatives of those involved to be accommodated away from the department as the large numbers that may be involved will be disruptive. Similarly the media should be catered for elsewhere, and ideally the department should be closed to all but staff and disaster casualties by the police. Routine casualties should be informed of the situation and told that they will have to wait a long time before being seen due to the disaster (assuming their clinical condition will permit of such a delay) and advised to go to another hospital or their GP. The notion of attempting to operate a non-disaster A & E unit in tandem with a department on major disaster plan is clearly a non-starter and will only result in sub-standard care for everybody. Liaison with the ambulance service is essential so that as far as possible 999 calls may be routed to another department.

Action cards for staff which describe their various functions are an excellent idea for it is likely to be quite chaotic preparing to receive casualties if different groups of staff are all trying to read through the same lengthy copy of the plan in an attempt to find 'their bit'.

Once the first casualties arrive, the need is for triage. This means sorting the casualties into categories so that those who need the care first, get it first and are not delayed by either less urgent cases, or more problematically, those who will die whatever care they are given. This needs considerable expertise and the senior nursing and medical staff on duty will need to be involved in this function.

There should be provision for a team from the hospital to go to the site of the disaster and it would seem logical that the A & E unit should provide the staff for this team because of their expertise in the trauma field. The team should be equipped with weather-proof clothing that for safety reasons is brightly coloured, including fluorescent tabards marked 'Nurse' and 'Doctor'. There should also be helmets with lights and Wellington boots in a full range of sizes. Equipment should be carried in backpacks rather than in one big trunk that may be impossible to carry near to the site of the disaster, although a back-up trunk containing reserve equipment is worthwhile.

The functions of the mobile team are two-fold: first to provide life-saving measures where appropriate and also pain relief for patients whose evacuation is not immediately possible, and second to carry out triage on-site.

To carry out the first function, equipment will be needed to secure and maintain an airway and breathing (including chest drainage), to set up IVIs, to dress wounds, to protect the injured from hypothermia (space blankets) and to give pain relief. The only surgical pack that is worth including is an amputation set and saw, together with the means to give quick-acting IV anaesthesia.

On-site triage is needed to insure that the most appropriate casualties reach hospital first. Theoretically this may mean that patients with probably non-survivable injuries such as 80% burns or bilateral high traumatic amputation of legs should be put to one side, in order that other patients go to hospital first, and treated symptomatically with analgesia only. In practice in a civilian situation, this would be very difficult to do, but if the scale of the disaster were big enough, it would have to be done.

A second function on site is that of splitting up the case load so that the ambulances distribute the casualties among the various departments in the area. This may not be possible in a rural area where there may not be more than one department within 30 miles, but in urban areas this is possible and greatly to be desired. In the Harrods bombing, St Stephen's Hospital received 39 casualties and the Westminster Hospital 37, a good example of sharing the workload.

One final point is that there is a high probability that casualties from a disaster will be suffering blast and high velocity missile wounds (shrapnel). These are injuries that are not covered in conventional nurse training. It therefore beholds authorities to insure that A & E staff are taught how these wounds and injury patterns differ from other forms of injury.

Not only should plans be constantly re-examined, but they should also be tested at least once a year to familiarise staff, and also to try and learn lessons that will allow further improvements. Such exercises allow for the building-up of liaison with the other emergency services which is so vital if the real thing ever happens.

Radiation Casualties

Many people are as afraid of radiation as they are ignorant of it and this includes nurses. Radioactive materials have played an increasingly important role in our way of life over the last 40 years and seem set to do so for the future. So although there have been few incidents involving radioactive materials so far, the possibility remains that one day an A & E unit is going to be confronted with a patient who has been involved in such an accident, and possibly many more than just one patient.

Atoms consist of a central nucleus composed of a cluster of positively charged particles (protons) and particles with no charge (neutrons), all held together by very strong forces. Surrounding the nucleus is a cloud of negatively charged particles called electrons that are almost one two-thousandth the mass of a proton and whose number equals that of the number of protons. The atom is, therefore, electrically neutral. Neutrons and protons are similar in mass, and the number of neutrons in the nucleus of a given element can vary, giving rise to the different isotopes of that element. The chemistry of an element is defined by the number of electrons orbiting the nucleus—from one in the case of hydrogen, two for helium, through to 92 in the case of uranium—and the number of protons in the nucleus, which should be the same.

This account of atomic structure is a great simplification, but it will suffice for our purposes. The effect of ionising radiation is to knock out an electron from an atom or molecule, leaving it with a surplus positive charge; in this state it is known as an ion. Radiation damages cells in the human body most commonly by forming water radicals—hydrogen atoms or hydrogen–oxygen atom combinations, with an electron missing. They are written as H^+ and OH^+ and are more correctly called ions. This occurs by the radiation knocking electrons out of water molecules in the cells. These radicals can chemically oxidise and destroy parts of the DNA molecule, disrupting normal functioning of the cells (Jankowski, 1982).

The effect on the human body of radiation will depend upon the energy of the ionising radiation, the frequency with which it will ionise atoms and molecules (knock out electrons), and its penetrating power. Table 21.1 summarises the penetration potential of the different forms of radiation that we may encounter.

In practical terms the penetrating power of α rays is such that they are unlikely to go beyond clothing or the outer layers of skin, while β rays penetrate only a few millimetres of tissue. Other forms of radiation,

Table 21.1
Summary of common forms of ionising radiation

Radiation type	Nature of Radiation	Penetrating Power	
		air	body tissue
α ray	Particle stream, each particle consists of two protons, and two neutrons.	6 cm	< 1 mm
β ray	Stream of electrons.	5 m	< 2 cm
x rays	Energy released by electrons changing position in atom.	10–100 m	whole body
γ	Energy released by nuclear particles reorganising position.	100+ m	whole body
Neutrons	Stream of neutrons.	100+ m	whole body

NB. The penetrating power of γ rays and neutrons is such as to make wearing lead aprons as used for radiology of little use.

while causing fewer ionising events for a given length of track, do however fully penetrate the body and therefore are able to damage rapidly dividing cells such as the cells in the bone marrow (blood-forming tissue) and in the lining of the gut.

The amount of energy in radiation is measured in rads (there are new units called grays, 1 Gy = 100 rad) while the amount of absorbed energy dose in human tissue is measured in rems (new units, Sieverts, 1 Sv = 100 rem); for practical purposes 1 rad equals 1 rem in most cases. The effects of an absorbed whole body dose of ionising radiation are described in Table 21.2.

In dealing with the real situation in A & E, the likely scenarios that we would encounter are that there is a patient who has been exposed to ionising radiation, or has ingested and/or inhaled radioactive material or has radioactive material on their body, with or without conventional trauma in each case.

A person who has been exposed to ionising radiation, but not contaminated with radioactive material, is *not* radioactive and therefore not a danger to anybody else. The damage has been done, just as somebody who has been shot is no longer a danger to anybody else: the bullet has done its damage and gone, the ionising radiation has gone. They may be treated in the normal way in A & E, but will need special in-patient care

Table 21.2
Effects of radiation—radiation sickness syndrome

Whole Body Acute Radiation (Exposure in Rads.)	
0–150	Either no symptoms or generally unwell and nauseated. Significant fall in blood lymphocyte count.
150–400	Bone marrow disease. Days 1–2 after exposure: unwell, nausea and vomiting. Weeks 2–3: fever, skin haemorrhages, mouth ulcers, loss of hair at more than 300 rad. Marked fall in blood count with maximum bone marrow depression at 30 days.
400–1000	Enteric disease. Day 1: unwell, nausea and vomiting. Weeks 1–2: fever, profuse bloody diarrhoea, loss of gut lining. Week 3: bone marrow disease if still alive. At 400–450 rads, 50% mortality for young fit adults. At 600 rads, near 100% mortality.
1000– plus.	Central nervous system disease. Lethargy, unsteadiness convulsions, coma and death within days.
4000–plus.	Death in a matter of hours.

Based on data in BMA report, *The Medical Effects of Nuclear Weapons* (1983), and after Hartog M., Humphreys J., and Middleton H. (1981) *Medical Consequences of the Effects of Nuclear Weapons*.

depending on which aspect of the radiation sickness syndrome develops according to the absorbed dose. Regular blood counts are required together with antibiotics and blood transfusions, consideration being given to the need to barrier nurse the patient in view of their lowered resistance to infection.

If a person is contaminated, urgent life-saving measures must take priority over decontamination otherwise the result may be death.

The basic principles of reception and treatment in A & E are to decontaminate the patient; to prevent the spread of contaminated material around the unit by isolation and by reducing the number of staff involved to the minimum; to protect staff looking after the patient; and to obtain monitoring equipment and personnel from the hospital physics department. Protective clothing such as plastic gloves and aprons should be worn but they will not prevent radiation affecting staff; they will simply prevent skin and clothes becoming contaminated with radioactive material. Conventional injuries should be treated as far as possible

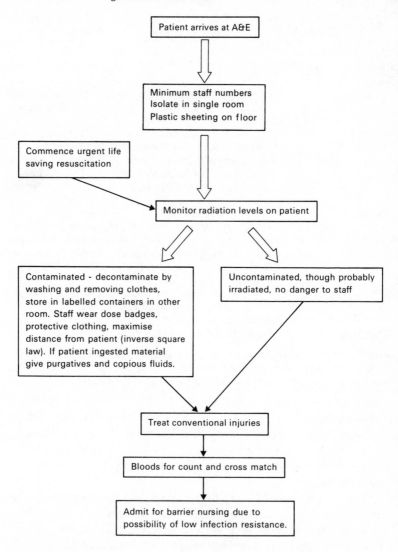

NB. Inverse square law means that the intensity of radiation decreases inversely with the square of the distance. Therefore by doubling your distance from the patient, you reduce the radiation intensity to one quarter of previous level.

Fig. 21.1   Flowchart for radiation casualties in A & E.

in the normal way, with great importance attached to psychological support for the patient. (See Fig. 21.1 for the sequence of management.)

A & E staff may find themselves asked about civil defence planning for war, especially since the recent appointment of planning officers to Regional Health Authorities to make Regional plans for the NHS in time of war. A series of reports by the RCN, BMA and World Health Organisation (WHO), all published in 1983, concluded that to try to plan for the effects of a nuclear war is impossible as the magnitude of casualties, both conventional and radiological would be so vast and the disruption to the infrastructure of society so great, that there would be nothing left for the survivors to do except sit and shiver in their nuclear winter and envy the dead. The scale of the problem is summarised by Openshaw and Steadman in their paper delivered to the 1983 conference of the Institute of British Geographers and quoted in the BMA report. Looking at a typical counterforce attack pattern against the UK, Openshaw and Steadman predict over 40 million deaths. The RCN report, looking at the effects of a single 1 megaton airburst over the city of Bristol, estimates that only 100 hospital beds would survive on the periphery of the city in cottage hospitals and that only about 325 nurses would be expected to survive and be reasonably fit; the number of casualties would be of the order of 100 000 with approximately twice as many killed.

A & E nurses are recommended to have nothing to do with the Walter Mitty world of Civil Defence planners. There are far more relevant and realistic issues for nurses to devote their time and energy to in the field of A & E nursing.

References and Further Reading

BMA (1983). *The Medical Effects of Nuclear War*. London: BMA

Hartog M. *et al.* (1981) *Medical Consequences of the Effects of Nuclear Weapons*. Cambridge: Medical Campaign Against Nuclear Weapons.

Jankowski C. B. (1982) Radiation Emergency, *AJN*. January. pp 90–98.

Nursing Times (1984). The Harrods Bombing (news report). *Nursing Times*, **80:3**.

RCN (1983) *The Consequences of Nuclear War Civil Defence Planning for Nurses*. London: RCN.

WHO (1983) *Effects of Nuclear War on the Health and Health Services*. Geneva: WHO.

Chapter 22

NURSING RESEARCH IN A & E

Why Research in A & E?

The last chapter in a book is often in the nature of a postscript. However, this book will not end with a look-back or an added-on afterthought, but rather with a look forward at an opportunity for the development of A & E nursing. That opportunity is nursing research.

One of the distinguishing features of a profession is thought to be a discrete body of knowledge distinctive to that profession. If nursing is to be regarded as a profession, then it must be based on a body of nursing knowledge, rather than on bits and pieces of knowledge taken from medicine. Certainly there is a need for close links with the various other professional groups in the health care field, and much can be learnt from them, but nursing also needs to develop its own body of nursing knowledge.

One way of acquiring nursing knowledge is simply to do what we have always done, which is to pass procedures (often with no sound basis) on from generation of nurses to generation as either revered traditions or mystical truths beyond question. But if other areas of human endeavour had followed that method, then it is likely that we would still believe that the earth is flat and at the centre of the Universe and that people who talk of wheels are dangerous disruptive elements or simply mad.

Human knowledge has advanced through questioning and enquiry, through reason and experiment, i.e. research, and so it should be with nursing. That is why there is a need for nursing research, carried out by nurses, and in a specialist field like A & E, there is a need for A & E nursing research to supplement that done in other fields of nursing.

How Do You Carry Out Research?

Polit and Hungler (1983) describe two basic research designs, experimental and non-experimental. In the former case the researcher studies the effect of some action or manipulation, e.g. a new wound dressing; in the latter case, no physical act is involved, but rather we are concerned to gather information about a problem or behaviour either by a survey or observation.

Another way of looking at research is to consider the method employed. We can either start off with an idea that we wish to test by research to see if we can find evidence of support or not. This idea is called a hypothesis and the method, a hypothetico-deductive method. A hypothesis cannot be said to be proven or disproven by research. Those statements are too definite given the potential for error and uncertainty that exists even in the best designed experiments. Instead we should talk in terms of a supported or a not supported hypothesis. The hypothetico-deductive method lends itself to either an experimental or survey design, and requires careful statistical analysis of its findings.

An alternative method is to start off not with a clear idea or hypothesis that we wish to test, but rather with an interest or problem that we wish to investigate. The researcher then sets about gathering information by observation and unstructured interviews, from which it is possible to make certain statements that the gathered evidence tends to support. This is the inductive method and has the advantage that as you did not start out with a definite idea, there is less chance of bias creeping in along the way as you try to confirm the idea that you suspect to be true.

In order to carry out a research project, the nurse needs to decide which method to use—the hypothetico-deductive or the inductive—according to the nature of the problem. (Is he or she testing a definite idea or just generally looking at a problem area?) Having selected the *method* that is appropriate, it then remains to select a *design* which is appropriate—experimental, survey, observational or a combination of different designs.

Experimental Research

True experimental research involves a manipulation, and that which is manipulated is known as the independent variable, the observer noting the effect of this on the other variable, the dependent variable. For example, in a wound healing experiment, the type of dressing applied is the independent variable and the rate of observed healing would be the dependent variable, i.e. it depends upon the dressing.

A second ingredient of an experiment is that there must be a control, a comparison group which is not subjected to the manipulation or act that is the subject of the experiment, so that the effect of the manipulation can be fully assessed. In nursing, we could not withhold nursing care in many situations to see how our control group compared with the group upon whom we tried out our new dressing, but Polit and Hungler consider that having a control group of subjects who receive the conventional dressing or treatment that was in practice before the new treatment under investigation, constitutes a valid control.

Randomisation constitutes the third essential part of a true experiment. This means that each subject has an equal chance of being in either group, experimental or control. This is essential to eliminate bias. Where relatively small groups are used, it is essential to match certain characteristics such as sex and age, as otherwise substantial distortions can occur by chance inclusion of a disproportionate number of a certain type in a group.

In many practical situations, it is not possible to rigorously fulfil all these three criteria of a true experiment. Techniques are available to overcome the problems of lack of full control or randomisation which still permit the findings of the research to have meaning. This is known then as quasi-experimental research and the reader is referred to Polit and Hungler for an account of these techniques.

Survey Research

In practice it is usually impossible to try to obtain information from every single member of the population that you wish to investigate (that would be a census), so the researcher has to use a sample of the population, a smaller group which to be acceptable has to be truly representative (contain the same proportions of characteristics as the total population in terms, for example, of sex, age and occupations) and has to be randomly selected.

The information may be gathered from questionnaires, although they have to be very carefully constructed so as not to lead the subject into answers. The wording of the question also needs careful attention as what may be obvious to the researcher phrasing the question may not be obvious to the subject trying to answer it. Another method of gaining information is the structured interview in which the researcher has a questionnaire worked out in advance and interviews the subject in order to gain the information. This eliminates misunderstanding of questions and other problems such as whether the person to whom the questionnaire was sent actually fills it in, but it does introduce an element of interviewer bias, although this can be minimised to some extent by close conformity with the questions as though it were a script.

Observational Research

This is sometimes known as ethnographic research, and is useful for studying subjects such as communication behaviours, activities and the characteristics of individuals and the environment. The interaction between the observer and the observed is vital as it can distort the observed behaviour and is fraught with ethical problems. Information is obtained by passive observation, participation observation and by unstructured interviews. Recording of data is carried out by various methods such as checklists, rating scales and tape recorders, all of which have advantages and disadvantages.

What Can be Researched in A & E?

After this brief introduction to some of the methods and terms involved in research, it is hoped that the A & E nurse may already be able to recognise problems in A & E that are amenable to research.

Take the example of complaining and aggressive behaviour from patients. This could be studied by the observational (ethnographic) approach, or experiments could be designed to try and reduce aggression (staff training, a TV in the waiting area), or a survey could be carried out of a sample of departments in the UK to test whether aggressive behaviour is worse in urban areas. Patient expectations, student nurse teaching and experience in the department, wound treatments, causes of accidents, and cost-cutting measures are all examples of the sort of problems that are amenable to nursing research and where the result would be an addition to the store of nursing knowledge and better treatment for our patients.

The limit of nursing research opportunities in A & E is the limit of your imagination and that of your managers. Research is not the sole province of a few academics in university departments of nursing, but rather should be the concern of nurses at clinical level, for that is where the results of research should be applied to ensure better nursing care. If A & E nursing is to develop fully in the professional sense in the years ahead, then it needs to be based upon sound research.

References

Polit D., Hungler B. (1983). *Nursing Research: Principles and Methods*. Philadelphia: J. B. Lippincott Company.

Cormack D. ed. (1984). *The Research Process in Nursing*. Oxford: Blackwell Scientific Publications.

INDEX